Kathy,

Thanks for all that you do for us and for people in general?

Jim Power
6/29/07

YOUR HEALER WITHIN

YOUR HEALER WITHIN

A UNIFIED FIELD THEORY
FOR HEALTHCARE

Dr. James McGovern
Dr. Rene McGovern

Fenestra Books

This book is dedicated to the readers who will enrich their lives and the lives of others by acting upon it.

Your Healer Within: A Unified Field Theory for Healthcare

© 2003 by A. T. Still University
All rights reserved. Published 2003

Publisher's Cataloguing-in-Publication Data

McGovern, James.
    Your healer within: a unified field theory for healthcare /
by James McGovern, Rene McGovern
    p. cm.
    Includes bibliographical references and index.
    LCCN: 2003103878
    ISBN: 1-58736-199-X (hardcover)

    1. Medicine—History. 2. Osteopathy. 3. Healing—History.
4. Still, A. T. (Andrew Taylor), 1828-1917. I. Title.

RZ321.M34 2003   615.5'33'09

Published by Fenestra Books™
610 East Delano Street, Suite 104,
Tucson, Arizona 85705, U.S.A.
www.fenestrabooks.com

Cover design and interior illustrations by Jamie Carroll
Book design by Atilla Vékony

Printed in the United States of America

CONTENTS

Chapter VIII

Chapter IX

FOREWORD

THIS IS a powerful little book. James and Rene McGovern have interpreted history from ancient times to today from the standpoint of individual health. From their sweeping review of historical writings by philosophers, healers, and scientists from around the world, emerges a confluence of cultures—European, Asian, Muslim, Buddhist, and Jewish—and a reconciliation of ancient and modern views of health and illness. The ultimate messages are that mind, body, and spirit are interconnected and that healthcare professionals must take all three components into account in order to render effective treatment.

These are essentially the same conclusions articulated by Andrew Taylor Still, a late nineteenth and early twentieth-century physician who was the founder of osteopathic medicine. In an effort to examine the philosophy and scientific basis for Still's writings, the authors realize that a lot of what we think of as new trends in healthcare—so-called "alternative" or "integrative" medicine, relaxation therapy, and the like—really have their roots in ancient times, in many cultures, and in scientific research. And most strikingly, Andrew Taylor Still saw all those connections and developed a new approach to medicine.

Osteopathic medicine thus emerges as an approach to healing with strong roots in humanism, psychology, and physiology, and one that takes account of the powerful ability of the human body to heal itself, hence the book's title, *Your Healer Within*. Emphasizing concerns for the whole person, rather than biological reductionism, and drawing on the scientific methods of observation and experimentation, this book ultimately provides a blueprint for physicians and other healers.

After reading this book, one is convinced that health and healing derive from complex interactions not only within bodily systems but also between the mind, body, and spirit. We are reminded that listening to patients is vital to understanding illness and affecting the healing process. We are awestruck at how close to the truth many of the ancient philosophers and healers came through simple observations, which have subsequently been confirmed by modern science. The McGoverns have brought all these threads together in a scholarly and readable book that will be of interest to health professionals and lay people alike.

Marian Osterweis, Ph.D.
Washington, D.C.

OVERVIEW

All perception of truth is the detection
of an analogy.

—Henry David Thoreau

PREFACE

THROUGH the centuries, physicians, scientists, philosophers, and thinkers of all kinds have pondered the body's amazing healing ability. Some have sought to go beyond the physical to examine the mental and spiritual aspects of healing. This book unites the collected wisdom of many ages, cultures, and fields of study with modern research findings. In most cases, theorists provide insights in their original words so that their messages would not be misinterpreted. Ultimately, this book pursues a set of principles that can provide an overall *context* for different approaches to healthcare.

The motivation for this book began with the extraordinary writings of Andrew Taylor Still, M.D., D.O., the founder of the osteopathic medical profession. In his numerous papers, articles, and books, Still promoted a revolutionary holistic approach to healthcare. His basic concepts are still valid today and are the key to coordinating the various approaches to healthcare. We shall see how his concepts answer the questions of *who, what, how,* and *why* in healthcare analysis and treatment.

Today, the osteopathic profession has grown to include twenty osteopathic medical schools. The increasing popularity of these schools is attributed to their emphasis on treating the whole person: body, mind, and spirit. Apparently, today's applicants know enough psychology or have enough experience to understand that healing, and hence medical education, should involve the interactions of the body, mind, and spirit.

How did a country doctor, practicing in the heartland of America in the second half of the nineteenth century, develop such a comprehensive treatment system? Our only clue is that he continuously asked for medical books and claimed that he read everything on healthcare from the early Greeks to his own times. In investigating Still's philosophy, it is curious that he seemed to derive lessons that differed from the traditional interpretations of some great medical philosophers. This sparked an investigation into some of the original works of Hippocrates, Galen, Virchow, Pasteur, Darwin, and others. Not only was Still accurate, but the popular explanations of these same items seemed to have missed the essential points.

This book is about understanding, sometimes for the first time, the true meaning behind some of mankind's outstanding medical discoveries. It is also about one of the greatest syntheses of medical history, where Andrew Still integrated some of these past insights into fundamental principles.

This book examines findings from several fields of study, including recent research, in order to provide an overview of healthcare approaches from Ayurvedics and Buddhism to approaches like the Relaxation Response and Naturopathy. Such coordination has been increasingly sought as physicians and others trained in traditional medicine have found themselves limited in their response to patients who have turned to herbs, meditation, and other Eastern or alternative approaches to care. Therefore, this book should prove helpful to health professionals and people in general who are searching for a basic, overall understanding of health-care.

The book follows an inductive process of seeking generalities among several cases. It gradually unfolds key insights and allows readers time to arrange them in their own way. As people put relationships together in their own ways, their brains form linkages that can be used to recall, rearrange, and derive further relation-ships. While learning is an individual process, we shall see that the laws of nature, including those about the human body, mind, and spirit, are interrelated. We shall also see that these relationships are elusive.

We are about to begin a quest together across the findings of several centuries. The people referenced are among the finest intellects in the history of mankind. While they have made definite contributions to our final model, the various healthcare approaches (Ayurvedics, Chinese Medicine, Naturopathy, etc.) and the various treatments (group networks, pet therapy, relaxation, etc.) discussed are not individually signifi-cant. These were chosen among many possibilities to illustrate how our model and theory could be univer-sally used.

Today, large numbers of self-help and health-improvement books are published every month. This book can provide a unifying context for the various approaches and treatments. Also, this book should be *personally* useful. As such, this book may be read for both personal improvement and the improvement of others.

Let us begin, keeping an eye open for useful analogies that Thoreau said are as close as we can get to truth.

James McGovern, Ph.D.
Rene McGovern, Ph.D.
Kirksville, Missouri

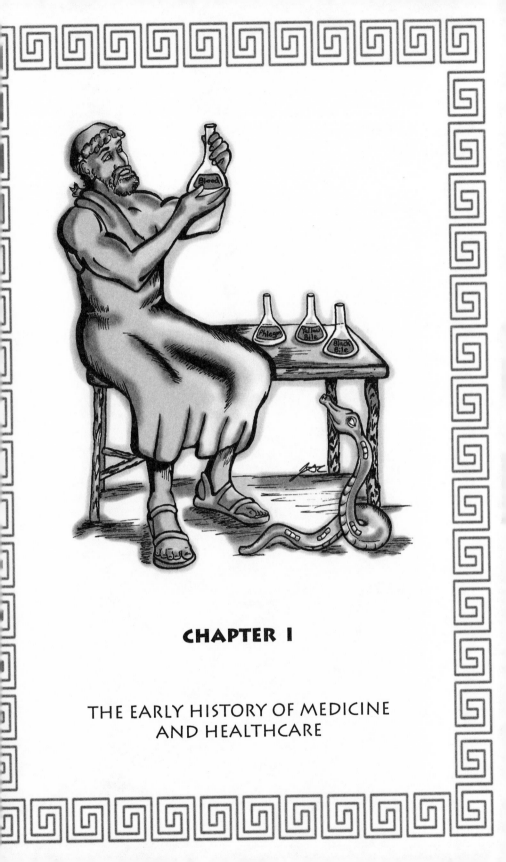

CHAPTER I

THE EARLY HISTORY OF MEDICINE AND HEALTHCARE

THE EARLY HISTORY OF MEDICINE AND HEALTHCARE

Those who know truth are less than those who appreciate it.

—Confucius

THIS CHAPTER provides a selective look at some key items in medical history. The goal is to present a brief look at the insights of a number of healthcare philosophers, and then draw from these sketches in later chapters.

Primitive Cultures

The story of medicine and healthcare is as old as the history of mankind. The first important lesson about primitive practices is that some of them seemed to work. When looking at chants, potions, bleedings, rituals, and other primitive approaches today, we conclude that many of them should not have worked. This suggests that there may be a large role for **auto-suggestion** in the healing arts.

The study of ancient medicine also illustrates that it was long on confidence and short on progress. That is, in every century and culture, healers confidently recommended "healthcare" procedures that were found later to be useless. However, the *extent* of efforts in seeking remedies was phenomenal. Perhaps the importance of health drove the continuous search for cures. Perhaps too, the effects of auto-suggestion encouraged the displays of confidence as a part of good practice.

In their earliest days, medical practices were filled with a mixture of myths, superstitions, and traditions. This mixture made it difficult to resolve the real causes of illness. Since many explanations of *how* health was restored were purely speculative with no physical measures, these myths could be repeatedly credited for cures with little fear of being proven otherwise. Thus, while speculation without possible measures may be beyond criticism, it is not useful for successively improving explanations.

The linkage of spiritual and physical aspects of illness is a prominent trend in early healthcare. The fact that aspects of well-being beyond the body itself have been discussed through the ages suggests that healthcare is multidimensional. Indeed, the focus on the body and the spirit in healthcare explains the linkage of healers and priests during primitive, medieval, and recent times. For instance, in ancient Egypt only priests were allowed to treat people.[1] Such historical facts can be worked back to the present to suggest that some aspect of spirituality may be needed or at least helpful in healthcare.

The study of the primitive history of medicine reveals that naturalistic and supernaturalistic approaches to healthcare have coexisted since the earliest days.

However, careful inspection reveals that their relative importance varied in a reciprocal way: when naturalistic medicine was in vogue, the supernaturalistic approach was in decline.[2]

While the study of medicine and healthcare practices over many centuries yields several general lessons, there are other more subtle lessons which are only detected by a closer, more detailed inspection. For instance, the fact that major discoveries are largely the result of *individual insight* is not noticed when we generalize over too wide or too distant a framework. The next sections feature individuals who made major findings about the mysteries of human functioning. Unfortunately, due to limitations of time and space, we can only discuss a few of the people who made contributions to the fundamentals of healthcare.

Choi of China (500 B.C.)

In Chinese medicine, the goal was to restore harmony with nature (*tao*). While the ancient Chinese developed many models to try to explain health and disease, including the linkage of specific emotions to specific organs, one of their most enduring models was their linking of pulse types with bodily ailments. To them, disease was a disorder in one or more organs and so pulses should be disrupted accordingly. In one treatise, ten volumes were needed to explain the wide number of pulse types that supposedly provided a comprehensive evaluation of the entire human body.[3] The various pulse types were given descriptive names like "willow breeze" or "bubbling brook" to help students and practitioners sort and remember them. In other words, language was important to the conceptualization and codification of differences.

The theory behind pulse types is that blood flows to and from all the organs of the body and abnormalities or problems in a particular organ cause particular variations in the circulatory system, which can be monitored by feeling the pulse. Feeling the wrist to get a "reading" on all the organs of the body was convenient in a culture that valued modesty. For instance, priests (physicians) sometimes felt the pulse of a woman through a curtain or provided a small doll to point to the part of the body that hurt.

A relationship between the variations of blood flow and problems in various organs was articulated by highly descriptive terms in order to form a comprehensive model for healthcare. In this example, we can also see how the prevailing customs or culture can "color" the types of models or procedures established. In other words, formulations use the thoughts, beliefs, and customs at hand.

Hippocrates of Greece (400 B.C.)

The works of Hippocrates come from the "Hippocrates Collection" gathered at the Library at Alexandria in Egypt at the beginning of the third century B.C. While no one can be sure that all, or any, of these books were actually written by Hippocrates, they were written during his time and were at the very least affected by his teaching.

Hippocrates was a teacher at the Aesculapian temple at Cos, which was named after Aesculapius whose existence is undetermined; he may have been a god, myth, or person. The important thing about these Aesculapian temples is that they were clinics or resorts where participants went to nurture their body, mind, and spirit. As has often been said: what was the *art* of Aesculapius became developed into the *science* of Hippocrates.[4]

Hippocrates, called the "Father of Medicine," removed the myths and superstitions from medical evaluations by relating causes and effects. Modern healthcare is indebted to him for proposing close observation and accurate interpretation of symptoms. He recognized disease as a departure from natural functioning and believed that natural laws could restore health if allowed to fully and properly function: "Natural powers are the healers of disease."[5] Hippocrates recognized four humors or attitudes and gave them bodily counterparts: blood, phlegm, yellow bile, and black bile. He said that health was when the humors were in proper proportions and disease was when they were not. He also believed that every person or case was different enough to disallow the possibility of accuracy in prescribing general medicines for individual people.

Hippocrates taught that medicines were secondary and exercise and diet were primary. As a Greek in a time of great philosophic awakening, he introduced logical analysis and suggested that prognosis, or projection of future developments, was the goal of the physician.[6] Hippocrates believed that the physician should work with the natural processes of the body. He made observations regarding the relationship between **structure** and **function** in the body and placed great emphasis on the spine and the musculoskeletal system.[7]

Hippocrates summarized his observations and diagnoses, forming a "language of medicine" that could be used and improved by others. Thus, rather than stating isolated speculations, Hippocrates started a system that was directly linked to observations and so its conclusions could be refined and improved by subsequent observations and analysis.

Aristotle of Greece (350 B.C.)

Aristotle is usually not associated with the development of healthcare. However, since this book deals with the philosophical developments of healthcare, Aristotle rightfully gets a central role. Called "the Philosopher" by Dante and most medieval scholars, Aristotle is generally considered the founder of the **scientific method**, a method composed of the alternate use of the inductive and deductive forms of logic. The scientific method has brought great discoveries for over twenty-three centuries. Unlike Plato, who taught that knowledge comes from within, Aristotle taught that knowledge comes from without, through the senses to the mind. He also taught that we should first obtain a general idea of phenomena and then investigate the particulars.[8]

Aristotle was able to reconcile the apparent disagreement among four previous great philosophers on the nature of causality. Causality answers the question of what caused something to happen. Thales taught that there was a material cause; some *thing* caused the change. Heraclitus said there was an efficient cause; some *doer* caused the change. Pythagoras said change was caused by a change in forms; some new *formulation* was responsible. Plato said that there was a final cause involved in every change; some *objective* was driving or causing the change. Aristotle explained that these four philosophers were each talking about just one aspect of a cause: the things involved, the doers, the formulations, or the objectives behind the change.[9]

Aristotle's pupil, Alexander the Great, who conquered a large part of Asia, sent back examples of the flora and fauna of each region conquered. These gifts allowed Aristotle to do an extraordinary amount of dissection on a large number of animals and to write about the similarities and differences among species. He wrote fifty books on comparative anatomy and natural history, describing such organs as the nerves, heart, blood vessels, brain membranes, stomach, and proposed models for their inner workings. Aristotle's books became the first books of the Library at Alexandria. His grandson Erasistratus joined Herophilus in dissecting hundreds of human corpses and greatly added to the knowledge of the body. Dissections were soon forbidden by religious authorities in both Egypt and Europe, ending progress in that direction.

Aristotle's famous aphorism was: "The philosopher should begin with medicine; the physician should end with philosophy."[10] It seems that Aristotle did not approve of unsubstantiated speculation. His definition of philosophy was based on gathering empirical data and deriving overall or ultimate causes (principles). This scientific methodology lay hidden for many centuries except for occasional rediscovery by such Westerners as Roger Bacon (13th century A.D.) and Francis Bacon (16th century A.D.), the latter making it accessible to medical researchers for the past 400 years. In summary, Aristotle's contribution to medicine and healthcare was giving mankind the methodology to learn and to accumulate knowledge. We shall see that he was also to make another comprehensive contribution.

Susruta of India (A.D. 200)

Susruta viewed himself as an elaborator of the ancient Ayurveda (science of life), which was supposedly inspired by Brahman.[11] The Brahmist believed that the physician had to be both theoretically trained and practically practiced, and that hygiene and diet were at least as important as drugs. Susruta's book *Collection* listed over 1,000 diseases and natural cures.[12]

Susruta managed to convince local leaders that dissection and surgery were appropriate. He developed many kinds of surgical instruments and wrote procedures for various operations. He had mnemonic names for surgical instruments that were related to their shapes, like "eagle," "heron," and "lion's jaw."[13] Surgery constituted the ultimate in Indian medicine and was, by its nature, free from speculation.[14] Surgery in India long remained beyond the reach of other nations.[15] The system of surgery remained at a high level of development in India for centuries and was founded on bold intervention, accurate diagnosis, and thoughtful after-treatment.[16]

Why was surgery so successfully developed in the early days of India and why did it eventually decline? While surgery is only a small part of healthcare, the answer to these two questions may be instructive to all parts of healthcare. The usual reason given to the success of surgery in India in the early centuries is that Indian governments punished criminals by ordering mutilations, and surgeons were then needed to repair these individuals.[17] On the other hand, the reason for the decline in Indian surgery may best be given by the following quotation:

Indian medicine was in possession of an impos-
ing treasure of empirical knowledge and technical
achievement; it reached to the height of a systematis-
ing, theorising school of thought, but it lacked the
freedom of individual action essential to the pursuit
of real science; it lacked too unprejudiced judgment
and the possibility of criticism, not stopping short
even of venerated doctrines. In the strange repressive
cultural conditions is rooted the destiny that was to
cut short the process of evolution and to lead to
scholastic petrifaction.[18]

While this section illustrates the importance of a
descriptive language to differentiate procedures or
instruments, its main takeaway message is that lack of
freedom can lead to petrifaction. Specifically, prejudice,
disallowance of criticism, and veneration of present
beliefs were reported as the seeds of self-destruction.

Galen of the Roman Empire (A.D. 200)

Coordination of medical theory and medical practice began under Hippocrates and came to be known as
dogmatism.[19] However, in Alexandria, dogmatism split
into two sects: one under the followers of Erasistratus,
who based their philosophy of medicine on *anatomical*
data, and the other under the followers of Herophilus,
who based their philosophy on *clinical* data.[20]

In Alexandria at that time, no sect could find a way
to reconcile the schools of thought on how the body
worked and thereby reconcile the two proposed causes
of disease or health. In Claudius Galen, medicine
attained a "Second Father of Medicine" and a major
reconciliation of theoretical and clinical knowledge
that lasted eighteen centuries.

Galen grew up in Pergamos in Asia Minor and studied at its Asclepieion (or Aesculapian temple), which was a health resort that attracted large numbers of pilgrim patients. Galen studied anatomy and physiology in several places, including Smyrna, Corinth, and Alexandria, before working on the wounded gladiators at Pergamos. There, he combined theory *and* practice, the teachings of Erasistratus and Herophilus:[21]

> As physician to the gladiators he had mostly to do with surgery, wherein he devised ostensibly new [clinical] methods (e.g., in cases of severe injury soaking the bandages with red wine to allay inflammation), but he was keenly observant of cases likely to add to his *anatomical and physiological* knowledge and he made careful use of observations upon athletes concerning dietetics and gymnastic exercises.[22] (emphasis added)

In other words, Galen realized that the approaches of Erasistratus and Herophilus were not contradictory but useful in different ways, having come from different viewpoints.

Galen's career brought him to Rome as the physician to Emperor Marcus Aurelius. This allowed him almost full time to write his many books. Combining his great theoretical knowledge of anatomy and physiology and his extensive clinical experiences with the gladiators, his books revolved around the concepts of the **structure** and **function** of the body: "The harmonious operation of organic functions can only take place, however, when the material structure is normal. . . . Diseases of the organs are caused by their alterations in structure. . . ."[23] "The application of these general ideas to the theory of health and disease called

. . . for direct investigation into the structure and functions of the human body."[24]

Galen followed Hippocrates in believing that the four humors caused four personality types. He also wanted to be able to predict what would happen next, that is, to have an accurate prognosis. However, his anatomical knowledge and his logical mind made him seek a solid foundation for prognosis. That is why he based his prognosis on clinical diagnosis.[25] He taught that final diagnosis should be reached through the elimination of possibilities. Thus, Galen wrote his books linking prognosis with diagnosis and, although wrong on many specifics, gave the world a healthcare philosophy that has proven so useful that it is the main approach to the practice of medicine to this day.

Avicenna of Persia and Maimonides of Spain (A.D. 1100)

Avicenna studied in the library of the sultan of Bukhara in Persia. He was a physician of wide learning who developed organizing structures of the Muslim religion by applying Aristotle's ethics to the teachings of the Qur'an (Koran). This inspired another physician, Maimonides of Córdoba, Spain, to develop similar structures or principles of the Jewish religion by also using Aristotle's ethics. In turn, after Maimonides' work was translated into Latin, Thomas Aquinas developed principles for the Christian religion based on Aristotle's ethical structures. Thus, three major world religions now have a common substratum of ethical principles. Can we have a common substratum of medical principles?

The fact that Avicenna and Maimonides were philosophers as well as physicians should not come as a surprise since they were both strong admirers of Galen, who encouraged the study of philosophy. Their philosophic bent allowed their books to link medical *effects* with *causes*. This linkage of cause and effect will be shown to be important.

Another significant element of their works is that they included both **body** and **soul** in their discussions of medical philosophy. Maimonides came to this by way of his teacher Averroës, who also taught him about Avicenna's works. Indeed, Muslim medicine contained the beginnings of an overall healthcare philosophy in its attempt to link clinical effects and diagnostic causes.

Avicenna's *Canon of Medicine* was a mammoth encyclopedia of five books which, when translated into Latin, was taught in Christian universities for several centuries.[26] Its size alone made it authoritative, but that may also have prevented further development. The West had to wait for independent thinkers like Leonardo da Vinci (d. 1519) to challenge the anatomy of the *Canon*, even though much of it was obviously wrong. Paracelsus (d. 1544) burned his copy of the *Canon* publicly in Basel, and in 1628, William Harvey said the section on circulation of the blood was wrong. By the time of Thomas Syndenham (d. 1689), many medical teachers made no reference to the Islamic physicians.[27] Nevertheless, these philosophers and physicians brought the teachings of Hippocrates, Aristotle, and Galen to western Europe and thereby allowed subsequent generations to have the clues necessary to further unravel the fundamental mysteries of the human sciences.

Formulation of Theories

At this point, we need to confirm what we have learned about the formation of medical theories to help guide us in our subsequent analysis of more recent medical theories.

The successful theories of the past required someone to have the inductive insight to discover a key relationship. For instance, the relationship may have been between pulse types and organ functioning, or between personalities (humors) and illness, or between diagnosis and disease. Someone had **to notice** a consistent variation between two things: a potential measure and a bodily problem.

The second step seen in our historical review was the formulation of a model or simple way to articulate the above relationships. The model may have been language about pulse types like "willow breeze," or clinical observations (as in Hippocrates' books), or the structure-function interactions (as in Galen's books). A model allowed its language **to link** a measure and a phenomenon.

The third step in forming a successful theory in the past seemed to be the ability to draw lessons and to predict further developments (prognosis). The ability **to learn** has been seen as the most important factor if we are ever to improve and accumulate knowledge.

Summary

In the review of ancient methods, we saw a repeated, but unconscious, use of auto-suggestion, or what is called today the placebo effect. This was related to a linkage of the body with the mind and spirit in many instances of healthcare. This holistic approach was most pronounced in the Aesculapian spas. In the writings of past healthcare developers, we saw various attempts at linking bodily measures with bodily functions and this was summarized in the last section on the formulation of theories. In particular, both Hippocrates and Galen linked bodily *structures* and *functions*, including attitudes and bodily functioning.

Aristotle was cited for his contribution of the scientific method and for his reconciliation of four predecessors' theories of change or cause:

1. Pythagoras — the formulations of change
2. Thales — the materials of change
3. Heraclitus — the "doers" of change
4. Plato — the objectives of change

In the next chapter, examples are given of biological theories in more recent centuries. The examples are different from the usual citations regarding some famous individuals. These obscure but important insights were fundamental to the intermillennial integrations of a largely unknown physician working in the American Midwest during the second half of the nineteenth century. We shall meet him and his extraordinary syntheses in the next chapter.

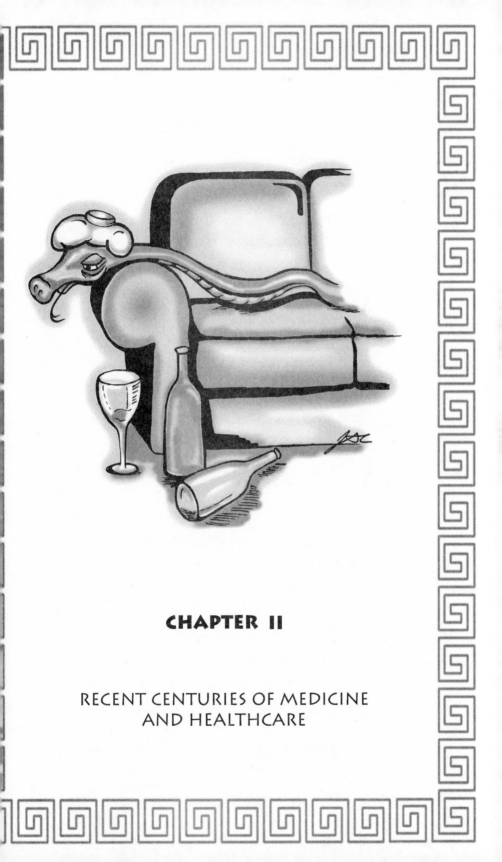

CHAPTER II

RECENT CENTURIES OF MEDICINE AND HEALTHCARE

RECENT CENTURIES OF MEDICINE AND HEALTHCARE

Such is the nature of truth that it only
wants its appearance.

—Thomas Paine

THIS CHAPTER discusses, in summary form, insights
of a few individuals in the last couple of centuries.
Some accomplishments may seem rather narrow, but
they will collectively move us toward a general understanding of healthcare.

Rush of the United States (A.D. 1800)

Dr. Benjamin Rush has been called the "Hippocrates of America" and the "American Galen," yet his
accomplishments are much more limited in quantity
and quality than these acclaimed predecessors. While
some people may think that progress is continuous, the
history of medicine shows that prevailing practices
have sometimes been retrogressive. The lack of historical insight has sometimes caused professionals to
repeat mistakes or to progress in circles.

Rush signed the Declaration of Independence of the United States and believed in freedom in several ways:

> The Constitution of this Republic should make specific provision for medical freedom as well as for religious freedom. To restrict the practice of the art of healing to one class of physicians and deny to others equal privileges constitutes the Bastiles [*sic*] of our science. All such laws are un-American and despotic. They are vestiges of monarchy and have no place in a republic.[28]

Rush became famous as a result of his work during the yellow fever epidemic in Philadelphia in 1762. However, this crisis made him believe that nature had to be controlled, or at least sometimes corrected. This philosophy of how medicine should be practiced is still held by many American physicians today.

Rush also worked in the mental health field and linked insanity to diseases of the brain. Ironically, he himself was charged with insanity in 1794.[29] He aroused quite a bit of opposition in trying to make reforms in Philadelphia. Even the board of health of the city of Philadelphia took an active part in opposing him.[30]

Rush was more appreciated after his death. While he only made a few improvements, he may have put a "slant" on medical practices that still exists in the United States. He is recognized for simplifying medical nomenclature, but he is best known for practicing "heroic" or interventive medicine. That is, instead of waiting for nature to act, he and many other American medical practitioners tended to intervene. They either did not trust nature or believed that they could do better.

Virchow of Germany (A.D. 1850)

The existence of cells had been known since the seventeenth century, but the development of new microscopes in the nineteenth century brought a new interest in the cell's role in healthcare.[31] In 1858, Rudolf Virchow published his book *Cellular Pathology*, wherein he claimed that the cells had to have good nutritional input and good waste removal.[32] Virchow pointed out a "body unity" where general health required that all the cells of the body had to be individually healthy since they were connected together.

Virchow concluded from his microscopic observations of cells that the various areas of each tissue depended on good blood-flow for nutrition and excretion and that various areas were somehow able to draw substances from the blood in order to obtain material for repair. Virchow concluded that a dysfunctional cell marked the beginning of disease.[33]

Pasteur of France (A.D. 1850)

Louis Pasteur was a chemist who explained the processes of developing different kinds of beers and wines; found a way to prevent milk from spoiling (pasteurization); saved the silk-worm industry; and found ways to deal with anthrax and rabies. His book on fermentation in 1857 was used as the basis of a new philosophy of medicine and healthcare.

Pasteur was asked to investigate why alcohol produced from beet juice was often contaminated. Using a microscope, he detected yeast along with another substance that later proved to be bacteria. He found that the yeast rotated polarized light, indicative of stereo-isomers, which only appeared in *living* substances. As explained later, he discovered that yeast are plant-like and bacteria are animal-like, suggesting microscopic flora and fauna.[34]

Pasteur's further experiments showed that he could control the amounts of yeast and bacteria by controlling the environment of acidity, heat, light, and so on. This is why different wines and beers have a variety of tastes; they are fermented (balanced) in different environments that produce various amounts of yeast and bacteria, yielding different tastes.[35]

Pasteur recognized that fermentation was respiration without air and could be part of a model to explain disease in animals.[36] Pasteur learned from his rival, Claude Bernard, that the body needed to maintain an ecological balance *(milieu interieur)* to control various living and chemical interactions.[37] The key question of healthcare then became how to maintain a healthy bodily environment (terrain) to keep the microscopic flora and fauna balanced and naturally controlled.

Today, most members of the medical profession follow Pasteur's concerns about bacteria and other germs, but overlook his advice about "balancing" their numbers within the bodily terrain. We have become a group of "microbe-hunters" rather than "micro-ecologists"; we are focused on killing rather than controlling germs.

Darwin of England (A.D. 1850)

Charles Darwin's writings on evolution and natural selection set the stage for a new sense of how nature works. Darwin believed that natural selection was the underlying mechanism under all the biological and medical sciences.[38]

Darwin's book *The Origin of Species* was sold out on the first day it was published in 1859.[39] Most commentators on his book have focused on the long-term (millennial) effects of the natural selections or internal optimizations that organisms make. However, Darwin also recognized short-term impacts that result from ongoing, daily readjustments:

> It may be said that natural selection is daily and hourly scrutinising, ... rejecting that which is bad, preserving and adding up all that is good; silently and insensibly working, whenever and wherever opportunity offers, at the improvement of each organic being in relation to its organic and inorganic conditions of life.[40]

In 2002, Stephen Jay Gould, Ph.D., of Harvard University, explained the central position of the interaction of structure and function in evolution in his book *The Structure of Evolutionary Theory*.

> An interactive model [is needed] to explain the sources of creative evolutionary change by fusing the positive constraints of *structural* ... pathways internal to the anatomy and development of organisms ... with the external guidance of natural selection (the *functionalist* approach).[41] (emphasis added)

Gould's explanation echoes the approaches of Erasistratus (internal, anatomical *structures*) and Herophilus (external, clinical *functions*) and their different attempt to explain bodily operations. Just as Galen reconciled the two schools of thought of Erasistratus and Herophilus into a structure-function interaction in the second century A.D., we shall next see how a man named Still integrated the insights of Virchow, Pasteur, and Darwin.

Still of the United States (A.D. 1900)

Andrew Taylor Still started a new type of medical school in Kirksville, Missouri, in 1892. Presently, the Kirksville College of Osteopathic Medicine is part of A. T. Still University. The impetus to start the school came from a visit in 1892 by William Smith, who had received his medical degree from Edinburgh University, one of the very best medical schools at that time. After spending much of the day watching Still treat patients and explain his theories, Smith said, "You have discovered that for which all [medical] philosophers have sought for two thousand years and have failed to find."[42] Thereupon, Still offered to teach Smith his principles and techniques, which he called osteopathy, if Smith would teach anatomy to the students in his new school. To assist them, Still hired a number of faculty including an M.D. from Harvard University, an M.D. equivalent from Glasgow University, and a Ph.D. from Columbia University; the last, John Martin Littlejohn (eventually the dean) also had medical and law degrees.

Still said his book *The Philosophy of Osteopathy* would "give to the world a start in a philosophy [of medicine and healthcare] that would be a guide in the future."[43]

> My object is to make the Osteopath a philosopher, and place him on the rock of reason. Then I will not have the worry of writing details, of how to treat any organ of the human body, because he is qualified to the degree of knowing what has pro-

duced variations of all kinds in form and motion [structure and function].[44]

Still believed that man had within him the remedies necessary to maintain health:

> When all parts of the human body are in line, we have perfect health. When they are not, the effect is disease. When the parts are readjusted disease gives place to health.[45]

As Still claimed to have read all the past medical philosophers, including the Greeks,[46] we can be fairly sure that he knew the works of Hippocrates and Galen, both of whom believed in the internal powers of healing and in the general sense that *structures* had to be in order so that *functions* could be in order. Wilborn Deason, D.O., once visited Still and observed him reading Rudolf Virchow's book about the cell. Still was intrigued by Virchow's observation that the health of the body was determined by the health of the individual cells, which depended on how well the cells obtained nutrition and removed waste. From this, Still realized how important it was to keep the various flows unobstructed in the circulatory, lymphatic, and nervous systems.[47]

Still also told Deason on that same occasion how useful he found the (Pasteur) theory of ferments or fermentation in the body.[48] Still explained that ecological structures could be used to explain why one person remained healthy while another obtained disease, i.e., when cells were able to ferment but not to remove waste. The "structure" of a cell was a living, dynamic system that had to be in order with proper inputs and outputs, if the body as a whole was to be able to function. From this, the importance of restoring bodily flows and nerve communication was deeply appreciated by Still:

> Dr. Still found that manipulation of the spinal column and its dependent tissues produced certain startling and special reactions, and this was strikingly the case whenever there was in the backbone any visible or palpable irregularity, lesion or deflection.[49]

Unlike previous medical philosophers who simply described models to *understand* bodily functioning, Still found a fundamental way to *liberate* the healing forces of the body:

> In Osteopathy not only was there an evolution but there was a revolution. Every system of treatment previously developed had been designed primarily to combat effects. Dr. Still's great work lies in the determination of cause, and through a knowledge of that cause, the application of an effective treatment.[50]

Still's many years of practice with bonesetting and spinal manipulations gave him an overall "map" of how the organs of the body were linked to various parts of the spine by the nervous system and between the heart and the circulatory system. Still then used **structure** and **function** to explain how the nervous, circulatory, and lymphatic *structures* had to be freed (by manipulation, for example) from constriction to allow them and all connected organs to *function*.

One osteopathic physician defined osteopathy as a part of evolution:

The fundamental law governing all existence—physical, chemical, vital, mental, and spiritual—is evolution. Evolution is marked by constant internal adjustment of the organism to its environment; to the physical, chemical, vital, mental, and spiritual forces playing on, in and through it.[51]

The evolutionary aspects of osteopathy came to Still through the works of Charles Darwin, Alfred Russell Wallace, and Herbert Spencer. These scientists recognized the ongoing self-healing process that was the natural selection or inclination of all living things. Andrew Still frequently referred to the concept of natural selection with the words "nature selects."[52] Still received the same overall philosophy from his father, Abram, who was a doctor and a Methodist minister. Methodists believed that self-perfecting was the duty of every human being, and so the concept of self-healing or perfecting in nature was an obvious belief for him. As a matter of fact, Still said that on June 22, 1874, he realized the main principle of osteopathy when it struck him that nature was always trying (evolving) to do its best at any given moment. This natural response is commonly known as natural selection, perfecting, or self-healing in the human body.

In conclusion, Andrew Still brought together the great insights of Virchow, Pasteur, Darwin, and Hippocrates to form the following fundamental principles:

1. **Interactive Unity**. The various parts of the body are interrelated, and disease or malfunctioning in one part can affect the functioning of other parts.

2. **Structure–Function Interdependency**. There are interdependencies between bodily structures and functioning; restoring natural structures helps functioning, and various types of functioning can affect the operating structures of the body.

3. **Self-Healing Mechanisms**. The body has a natural predisposition toward self-adjusting or adapting to restore natural structures and functioning.

4. **Holistic Treatment**. To be comprehensive in analysis and hence effective in treatment, all of the above basic principles should be considered.

Summary

A. T. Still's formulations of health and disease were based on biological theories and originally had nothing to do with osteopathic manipulation, which was developed later.[53] Still was basically trying to develop a *philosophy* of healthcare based on principles of nature.

Still used Virchow's sense of body unity among cells to formulate his principle of **Interactive Unity**, which holds that malfunctioning of one part of the body could affect the functioning of another part. Next, Still used Pasteur's sense of balancing the body's ecological systems or "dynamic structures" to form the basis of his principle of **Structure-Functioning Interdependency**. Thirdly, Still used Darwin's theory of natural selection or adaptation as the basis for his principle of **Self-Healing Mechanisms**.

1. Virchow — Interactive Unity
2. Pasteur — Structure-Function Interdependency
3. Darwin — Self-Healing Mechanisms

The principle of **Holistic Treatment** using the above three principles arose as a logical consequence of knowing these principles.

In the next chapter, we will learn about some of the subtleties within these healthcare principles. We will see that when aspects of the **mind** and **spirit** are included, these principles take on additional significance and insight. We will also see that health professionals have been seeking overall principles of healthcare for a long time. Some of these comprehensive principles have been buried in osteopathic principles with only a few commentators realizing their full potential.

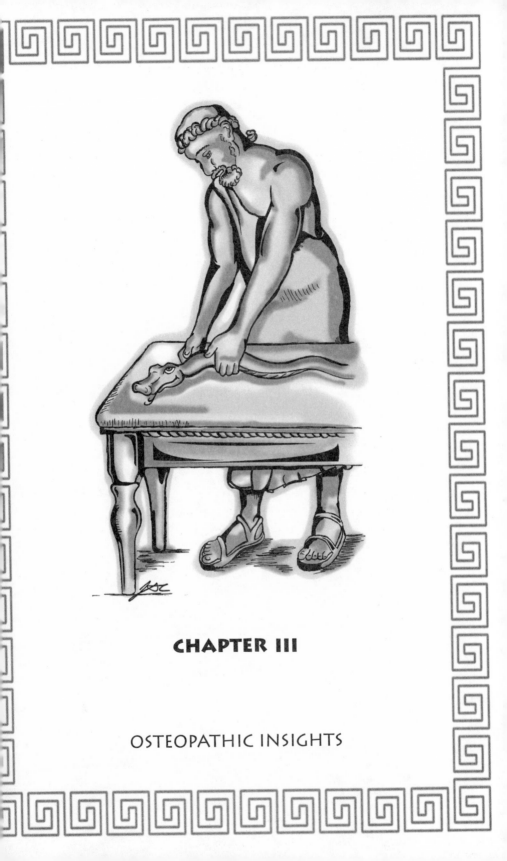

CHAPTER III

OSTEOPATHIC INSIGHTS

OSTEOPATHIC INSIGHTS

Metaphor is a tool for creation which
God forgot inside some of His creatures.

—Jose Ortega y Gasset

THIS CHAPTER further examines the principles of osteopathy. In particular, these principles are expanded to include the mind and spirit as well as the body. This chapter also brings together some of the great voices of the last century to describe why an overarching set of principles of healthcare is needed.

Drug Bust

Speaking generally, many physicians probably use medicines because their medical training taught that medicines were effective. However, long-term historical results point out the general ineffectiveness of drugs and suggest a belief system or psychological bias that *wants to believe in* effective drug treatment.[54] The belief that we can find the right drug or "magic bullet" lies deep in the human psyche and its tendency to believe in happy endings and man-made miracles. Therefore, we must not blame physicians *per se,* but instead blame human nature for the somewhat indiscriminate uses of medicines today and suggest that physicians and all healthcare professionals might be helped by having an overall healthcare philosophy of how the body (or whole person) works.

Of course, we are not questioning medications when a diagnosis indicates something is needed and the related medicine or inoculation has been proven effective over time. What we are suggesting is that today too many people assume that there is a medicine for every type of illness and want to take a pill or injection when it is not indicated by professional diagnosis or when the particular medicine has not been shown to be effective scientifically.

Some physicians—osteopathic (D.O.s) and allopathic (M.D.s)—believe that using drugs to treat disease without treating the underlying *cause* of the disease is a "hit or miss," or incomplete approach at best. Consequently, they believe that an overall causal model of bodily operations is needed. The following sections give a brief historical perspective to the development of a philosophy of healthcare based on the natural principles of cause and effect.

Still Wellness

In 1864, Andrew Taylor Still, a licensed physician, lost his three young children to meningitis in the span of a few weeks. He had been greeted by his children sitting in a window when he returned home each evening. He was so despondent about not being able to help his own children with the medicines of the day that he boarded up the window and gave up medicine for over a year.[55]

Eventually, Still used his personal loss to motivate himself to find new ways to help those with diseases. For over twenty-five years, from the late 1860s through the 1880s, he experimented with "bonesetting." He corrected structural aberrations in the bones, especially the backbone, and found that he could stop a large amount of dysfunction by returning the bodily structures to normal.

As Still worked with different impairments, he found that spinal and other musculoskeletal adjustments could cure many of the things he encountered. Since he started his analysis of pathologies by checking the structural integrity of the backbone, he referred to his treatments as **osteopathy**, since *osteo* was Latin for "bone."

Still likened body unity, or the coordination of parts and functions, to a machine. As a machine inventor himself, he was quite familiar with how machines relied on all the parts being in working order. The machine analogy gave him a simple causal model of how various systems had to interrelate in the human body. The spinal column, as a central structure, was highly important since it maintained a close relationship to the ganglia (nerve clusters) along it. In turn, these ganglia (including the brain) controlled all the parts of the body.

Still's development of natural principles and treatments brought hundreds of people to him in Kirksville, Missouri, in the 1880s and 1890s. Most significantly, he found a way to treat the fundamental *causes* of disease and not just address the *effects* of disease. Indeed, he explained that disease was a structural abnormality sometimes caused by an outside agent. When corrected, the body could return to its natural (healthy) state.

Still's machine or structural analogy gave the beginning of a way to understand bodily causes and effects.

Osteopathic Accomplishments

Good outcomes from osteopathic manipulation have been reported for over a century. However, given the small number of osteopathic physicians practicing a large amount of manipulation and the lack of scientifically controlled research, osteopathic manipulation has continued to be looked upon with suspicion. Because of the many dimensions involved and the wide variability among human beings, controlled experiments require large numbers to obtain statistical significance. Consequently, most endorsements for manipulation have been based on clinical, anecdotal testimony:

> When a given symptom disappears under spinal treatment alone it must have disappeared of its own accord or have been eliminated by the treatment. The duration and tendency of the symptom will decide which is the *more reasonable* of the two explanations. If the same thing occurs in several successive instances the relation is more firmly established. This is not proof but it is convincing evidence.[56] (emphasis added)

During the last century, osteopathic physicians have proven little through controlled research but have achieved apparent successes. During the height of the influenza epidemic in the early part of the last century, the *Chicago Evening Post* reported:

> Figures compiled by the osteopaths throughout the country show that out of 49,000 cases of flu

treated [by osteopathic manipulation], of which between three and four thousand developed pneumonia, only 472 died—a mortality of less than 1 percent. As nearly as can be estimated, the total mortality from flu thruout [sic] the country has ranged from 5 to 15 percent.[57]

Another study of one hundred cases treated osteopathically in a typhoid epidemic reported zero fatalities.[58] Other studies showed 76% success in the treatment of catarrhal deafness, 87% success with hay fever, and 80% with asthma.[59] In addition, a study on back problems in 1999, reported in *The New England Journal of Medicine,* showed osteopathic treatment to be at least as effective as medical treatments and notably less expensive.[60] These results suggest that there is at least some effectiveness in osteopathic manipulation and invite further study.

A. T. Still realized the underlying operational mechanism of spinal manipulations:

> It appears perfectly reasonable ... that all diseases are mere effects, the cause being a partial or complete failure of the *nerves* to properly conduct the fluids of life.[61] (emphasis added)

Specifically, Still believed that manipulation worked because the nerves stimulated bodily "drugs" and other internal responses to restore the body to natural functioning.[62]

Inner Meaning

Irvin Korr, Ph.D., of the Kirksville College of Osteopathic Medicine, further explained in 1962 the internal significances of manipulation:

Osteopathic manipulative therapy . . . is designed to eliminate critical impediments to the optimal operation of adaptive . . . processes. . . . It is a whole *system* [emphasis original] of diagnosis, appraisal, therapy, . . . subject to infinite variety of adaptations to individual requirements. Those influences cause the biologic—and therefore human—potential to be fully released, . . . in the cure that must come, if it comes at all, *from within.*[63] (emphasis added)

However, the focus on the natural healing processes *within* the body became increasingly unpopular during the twentieth century. Most of the training, and hence most of the treatment, during the century was aimed at finding specific drugs for specific "bugs." As Rene Dubos, Ph.D., of the Rockefeller Institute decried: "The doctrine of specific etiology [definite cause] had appeared to negate the philosophical view of health as equilibrium and to render obsolete the traditional art of medicine."[64]

Fortunately, osteopathy has consistently focused on the total person and on the healing by the forces within the person. A. T. Still generally, but comprehensively, defined *disease* as abnormal structure within the body and defined *health* as the absence of abnormal structures within the body. We will soon include psychological structures, or the inclusion of the whole person, in our discussions.

Trained with these general, natural principles, D.O.s have, in turn, treated patients fairly comprehensively during the last century. Osteopathic physicians were taught about the general sense of disease and health and realized that the power to heal lies within their patients, not themselves. They were educated about the need for the body parts to work together, using the nerves for communication and guided by the body's own self-healing responses. However, like all other healthcare professionals, osteopathic physicians still lacked an overall sense of how all the systems, including the psychological, worked together. There was not an integrative theory across the body, mind, and spirit, and hence treatment was partial and incomplete.

General Concepts Needed

More and more physicians and healthcare workers were looking for overarching structures to help comprehend the individual dynamics involved in both disease and health. In particular, they appreciated the need for an *overall* understanding. As Walther Riese, M.D., observed in 1953:

> Diseases, we were rightly taught, have to be related to their causes. But the postulate [above rule] implied the existence of *specific* causes which, to say the least, are as debatable today as ever.[65] (emphasis added)

The need for a comprehensive view of healthcare was also described by a long-time professor at the Kirksville College of Osteopathic Medicine, Harry Wright, D.O., in 1963:

> But now that medical thinkers are again reviving the view that health is essentially an equilibrium or harmony of action of the various organ systems of the body, the care of patients will undoubtedly demand a different type of physician in the future—a physician whose concern is focused on the patient rather than on local pathology. . . .

It appears that the role of the physician of the future will be more concerned with man and his environment—concerned with helping the individual to make the best possible adaptation to his environment. To do this he must consider not only the stresses, of whatever nature, in the patient's environment but the individual himself, his goals and aspirations in life. . . .[66]

As seen in the last few references, physicians have been seeking to find how, in general, self-healing worked within individuals. Hans Selye, M.D., of McGill University, came to the same conclusion that general principles were needed to articulate the natural healing within the body in the 1950s:

Throughout the centuries, we have learned virtually nothing about rational, scientifically well-founded procedures that would help the body in its own natural efforts to maintain health quite apart from the attacks on the pathogen. . . . Let us remember that it is not the microbe, the poison, or the allergen, but our reactions to these agents that we experience as disease.[67]

Selye gave a key insight to finding these natural, internal principles by defining disease as "our reactions." He was close to Still's definition of disease as our body's "abnormal structures," but Selye, who coined the word **stress**, knew that disease was caused by our reactions, which included those of the mind and spirit as well as those of the body.

Mind, Body, and Spirit Distinctions

Having established a fundamental sense of disease and health, it is now time to address the unity of mind, body, and spirit. A. T. Still believed in a unity or connectivity among the body and the mind and the spirit:

> Throughout his writings, Andrew Taylor Still emphasized that man exists as a total functioning unit and that one of the major factors in the preservation of that unit rests in the stability of the mind and its components.[68]

Just as there are internal and external assaults on the body of a person, there are internal and external assaults on the *mind* of a person. Similar to how we described bodily disease, we can describe psychological disease at this point. Our *unhealthy reactions* to stress, etc., can be considered to establish *unhealthy structures*, which can bring forth unhealthy mental functioning. Accordingly, we can have mental structures as well as bodily structures that affect related functioning.

Some healthcare professionals try to link specific stresses with specific mental disorders. However, physicians like Selye have suggested a more general cause of disease as did Still.[69] Disease can be considered as having poor or damaged structures, which can be mental as well as physical. These damaged structures can affect other parts of the person and, conversely, different parts of the person can cause problems with structures. That is, an interactive unity principle is at work in mental as well as physical parts of a person.

Some people can have various "disease agents" in their bodies and not succumb to illness; so too, people can have various stresses and not succumb to mental disorders. The answer to the paradox may be found in the osteopathic sense of disease and health. Health can be considered as having well-functioning internal mechanisms. These self-healing mechanisms work in helping mental functioning as well as physical functioning. Therefore, self-healing is at work for the mind as well as the body.

With this understanding, a person has a healthy or normal "structure" when in equilibrium with himself and the environment, and has an abnormal "structure" when there is dissonance. Therefore, stress can come upon some people and not cause illness because that person has natural (realistic) psychological structures. On the other hand, when one establishes unrealistic or unbalanced notions about oneself, abnormal or diseased structures develop wherein our self-healing mechanism cannot function properly.

The above overview provides a general context to the understanding of mental as well as physical disease and health. George Northup, D.O., reinforced these points in his 1953 article:

> Patients with what appear to be psychosomatic disorders seem to be reacting to emotional stresses and strains which are *no greater* than the stresses and strains being inflicted upon individuals who are clinically healthy. Therefore, it is my opinion that a person who is psychosomatically ill is not only triggered into his illness by a variable group of emotional factors, but is effecting a response which is *outside the limits* for his particular body unit.[70] (emphasis added)

The final area of the osteopathic treatment of mind, body, and spirit, is the *spirit*. Although A. T. Still had some keen insights into spirit, subsequent osteopathic physicians have sometimes misunderstood the spirit. Nevertheless, spirit has remained an integral part of their mind-body-spirit approach. For instance, most osteopathic physicians have addressed the drives and motivations of patients. Indeed, because of this wonderful tradition, they have asked patients about themselves, their fears, hopes, and beliefs about improving. From this personal approach to medical practice, D.O.s have learned that these "inner feelings" can be as much a cause of disease or wellness as abnormal or normal bodily parts can cause disease or wellness, respectively. They have also learned how to use these inner (usually unconscious) feelings *proactively* in treating both physical and psychological diseases.

Many physicians and other health professionals do not have a clear sense of the spirit or inner beliefs because they have not used words unequivocally to define concepts like conscious feelings, inner drive, belief, and will. Today, with so many books being written in these areas and using such words interchangeably, it is no wonder that there is so much confusion. Clarification will be part of the task of the next chapter. Suffice it now to say that the osteopathic principles need to be expanded to include the working of the mind and spirit, as well as the body, to properly consider the health of the whole person.

Summary

This chapter explained some of the implications of A. T. Still's philosophy of health and disease and began to unfold its implications in the areas of the mind and spirit. Disease was defined as an effect, as a result of disruption of a natural structure, including "structures" of the mind and spirit. The effectiveness of medicines was questioned, given their mixed history of success, and overall principles were urged. Various sources dur-

ing the past decades cited the need for general, nonspe-
cific principles to understand the body's coping
mechanisms. Toward that goal, osteopathic principles
of interactive unity, structure-function interdependency, and self-healing mechanisms showed wide application, even with problems of the mind and spirit.

Quotes from Still, Korr, and Wright pointed out the
highly comprehensive nature of osteopathic principles
where treatments of various kinds activated the nervous system (Still), activated the adaptive processes to
release the human potential (Korr), and considered not
only the stresses, but the individual himself, his goals,
and aspirations (Wright). This empowerment and activation of the individual's *natural functioning* is the essential message. As a result, a universal cause-effect model
of interaction among the mind, body, and spirit begins
to come into focus.

In the next chapter, we will introduce the concept of
a unified field theory and see how it can form the basis
for finding a unification across the fields of study of
the mind, body, and spirit.

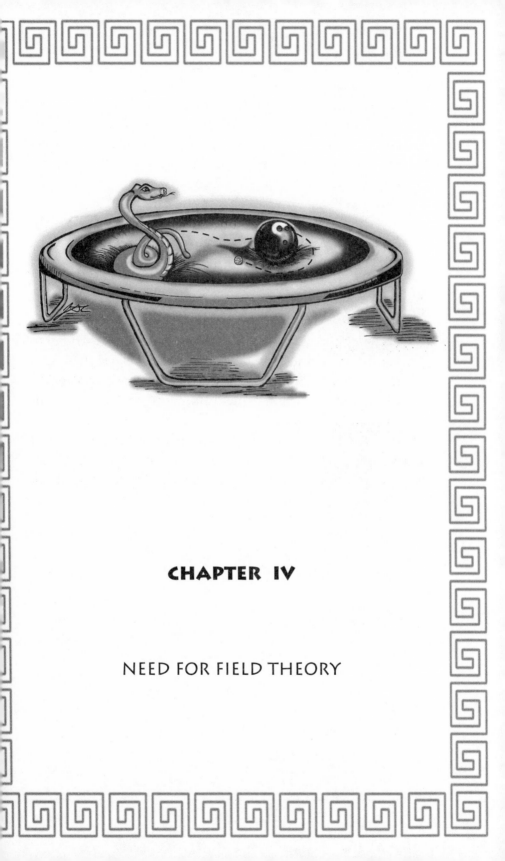

CHAPTER IV

NEED FOR FIELD THEORY

NEED FOR FIELD THEORY

Life is painting a picture, not doing a sum.
—Oliver Wendell Holmes, M.D.

THE MAIN call for an interactive theory has come from people like Hippocrates, Galen, Still, Selye, Dubos, and Riese. These individuals recognized that a single cause is seldom all that is involved in a complex human being, and that a general model was needed to link the various interactions of the body, mind, and spirit.

Unfortunately, the etiological approach of looking for specific causes for specific effects has dominated both research and treatment during much of the twentieth century. Of course, this narrow approach is important and forms the basis of the scientific method, but it is not always enough. We have to be open-minded enough to consider that an additional perspective may be helpful in giving us a model for understanding the causes and effects across the mind, body, and spirit.

Unified Field Theory of the Physical Sciences

Albert Einstein spent most of his life working on field theories. The last decades of his life were dedicated to trying to find a unified field theory which would link such areas as light wave propagation and gravitational forces. Experimental data showed that light propagation interacted with a strong gravitational field. This interaction between light and gravity showed that some kind of underlying continuity was involved.[71]

Explaining a gravitational field may serve to show how a field theory can summarize a large number of cause-effect relationships. For analytical purposes, Einstein said that matter seemed to "bend" space to the extent of its mass.[72] This can be envisioned if you place different objects on a trampoline or stretched membrane. A large man will indent the surface of the trampoline a lot more than a small child or ball. The small child or ball will tend to be attracted toward the man, just as in outer space the moon is attracted toward the earth. Fortunately, the moon also has tangential velocity, which is enough for it to fall, but fall around the earth. That is, the moon keeps falling beyond the horizon and so never reaches the earth.[73]

The above is the field theory of general relativity that summarizes millions of cause-effect equations and explains planetary motion around the sun and artificial satellite motion around the earth. In this case, the field theory happens to describe a field of action at a distance, but a physical field or surface is not necessary in order to have a field theory. In general, a **field theory** is a model that can simultaneously summarize many interactions of cause and effect and a **unified field theory** is a model that can summarize many field theories.

In the case of the gravitational field of the earth and the moon, the curved-space model allowed the National Aeronautics and Space Administration (NASA) to understand how an artificial satellite could escape the "slope" of the earth and "ride the curvature" of the indented space around the moon and safely return to earth. Similarly, such descriptive models may be able to help our understanding of people. We just need the openness to use general models, even if they describe "dynamic structures" or "curved space" that cannot be seen physically.

We have learned that theories should be able to link, predict, and teach. Since theories are only used by people, they are good to the extent that people find them useful in understanding (diagnosis), predicting (prognosis), and learning (practice).

In physics, good theories may not explain all exceptional cases but provide enough insight to be widely used and continued from generation to generation. It is hard to get any statement, and certainly any widely applicable theory, to be consistently true. So, with humility for imperfections, let us pursue a unified field theory for healthcare. However, before we do, we must first get a better sense of some of the interactions among the body, mind, and spirit. We have thus far only very generally introduced the structures and functioning of the mind and spirit in the last chapter. We will now continue the discussion of the mind and spirit, but this time we will include their interactions with the body.

Mind, Body, and Spirit Interactions

Although, A. T. Still did not truly integrate the treatment of mind, body, and spirit, he knew it was necessary for full understanding:

> We want to inform ourselves on that before we take hold of a man that has an enlarged liver [for example], because on the inner man depend the

results. . . . The spirit is the man, the inner man of whom I am talking.[74]

A fundamental sense of spirit resonates in the above quotation. In recent decades, the interaction among mind, body, and spirit has attracted a large amount of attention and so definitions are important before examining interactions in this area. In 1953, Cora Barden, D.O., claimed that physicians should link the **mind** with conscious psychology and the **spirit** with the unconscious psychology within a person.[75] The conscious mind is believed to control the voluntary nervous system, while the unconscious mind is believed to control the autonomic nervous system. Korr, in 1974, detected various autonomic muscular responses in patients disturbed by emotionally stimulating inputs.[76] Thus, there is empirical evidence demonstrating that the conscious mind is able to communicate with the unconscious mind. In addition, many other examples will demonstrate this interaction in later chapters.

It is important to distinguish between spirit and **belief** or **faith**. Belief may be defined as the assent by the unconscious mind to what has been declared by the conscious mind to be true. That is, the unconscious mind or spirit can come to believe a repeated, authoritative, or persuasive affirmation. This means that there can be healthy or unhealthy thoughts depending on how these affect our beliefs.[77] We should also realize from this discussion that healthy thoughts like hope, determination, and consideration can be transmitted to the spirit with or without a religious context. An affirming dialogue can produce belief if it occurs between a priest and parishioner, a doctor and patient, or a group leader and a support group. The goal is not just belief but a *healthy* belief so as to maintain a healthy spirit and thereby allow the autonomic nervous system and immune system to function properly.

The effects of the spirit, or unconscious mind, on health have been discussed for centuries. Hippocrates and Galen linked the humors or attitudes of patients with various kinds of maladies. In 1870, James Paget, M.D., described cancer predispositions as "deep anxiety, deferred hope, or disappointment."[78] In the last few decades George Vaillant, M.D., studied a group of Harvard graduates and found that those with good attitudes stayed healthy.[79] Similarly, recent studies of rheumatoid arthritis, lupus, and other autoimmune disorders show that the worse the disposition or semi/unconscious spirit, the weaker the immune system.[80]

In terms of the osteopathic principle of **structure-function interdependency**, the spirit needs to be in a healthy structure in order to function properly. That is, a person needs to have a happy or at least an open attitude to have a healthy framework for the mind and, hence, the body to function well. The mind, body, and spirit share the need for healthy structures. For instance, the body needs to have proper blood and nerve flows for the other parts, the mind and spirit, to function well. Osteopathy also provides the clue to *why* this happens: **interactive unity** causes one part to interact with other parts. Similarly, **self-healing mechanisms** operate in the mind (e.g., with conscious self-defenses) and in the spirit (e.g., with unconscious defense mechanisms) as well as in the body.

Further, each of these components (mind, body, and spirit) has subcomponents or aspects that affect aspects of the other two components. For instance, different types of nutrition can affect the body as much as their chemical reactions can affect various parts of the mind. Similarly, different emotional states can affect the various actions of the body. Indeed, one factor is seldom all that is involved:

> No single factor appears to be paramount in improving brain biochemical, cognitive, or emotional function. Instead, what emerges is a pattern of *multiple factors* related to an enriched environment that includes improved nutrition. This more comprehensive view of the nature-nurture debate concerning behavior results from the recognition that a converging **interface** [emphasis added] exists among psychology, neurobiology, learning theory, and nutrition.[81]

That is, while there is no single factor causing things to happen, the fact that many fields are involved suggests that an interface or continuity exists among the involved fields.

Unified Field Theory for Human Sciences

We will now try to put together a unified theory of these interactions in healthcare. It will be simple but also comprehensive enough to provide a useful framework.

After reading the previous sections, the reader can appreciate that the osteopathic principles of *body* unity, *body* structure-function interdependency, and *body* self-healing mechanisms could be expanded to include the total person with mind and spirit as well as body. That is, **Interactive Unity** can explain the unity of parts within the body, within the mind, and within the spirit. Similarly, with **Structure-Function Interdependencies** and **Self-Healing Mechanisms**, they can explain the structure-function relationship and self-healing in the mind and spirit as well as in the body.

But how do we explain the interactions *among* these three principles of osteopathy? We have three operational principles each separately explaining interactions of the mind, body, or spirit, but we have not expressed a basis of continuity *among* the principles *themselves*. In other words, what do these principles have in common?

Here is our discovery: these three principles align with the types of causes explained by Aristotle. That is, the commonality among these principles is that they are different types of causes. In other words, they are describing changes from three different viewpoints.

Aristotle said that each of the following philosophers was focusing on just one aspect of the cause of change:

Table I: Types of Causes

Philosopher	Type of Cause	Explanation
1. Pythagoras	Form(al) Cause	*How* did the forms (formulations) change?
2. Thales	Material Cause	*What* things have changed?
3. Heraclitus	Efficient Cause	*Who* ("doer") made the change?
4. Plato	Final Cause	*Why* did the change occur?

Comparing these different perspectives on causes to the osteopathic principles, we derive the following alignment:

1. The **form(al) cause** explains changes in terms of the formulations or concepts involved. This is

also the viewpoint of the principle of **interactive unity**. Interactive unity is one perspective on change when we want to focus on *how* things changed according to some concept or continuity across the changes.

2. The **material cause** describes changes according to the materials or structures involved. This is also the perspective of the principle of **structure-function interdependency.** Structure-function is another way to look at change when we want to consider *what* materials or structures changed.

3. The **efficient cause** portrays change in terms of the doers or processes involved. The principle of **self-healing mechanisms** also explains changes in this way. The self-healing mechanism is a third type of cause or third perspective on change that is instructive when we want to focus on *who* or the processes involved.

The following table summarizes these alignments:

Table II: Alignment of Causes and Principles (Incomplete)

Type of Cause	Explanation	Healthcare Principle
1. Form(al)	How did formulations change?	Interactive Unity
2. Material	What things have changed?	Structure-Function Interdependency
3. Efficient	Who made the change?	Self-Healing Mechanisms
4. Final	Why did the change occur?	(Forthcoming)

In summary, the continuity across the healthcare principles is that they are types of causes. The cause of something can be looked at in various ways: the formulations or conceptual models, the materials or structures, the doers or processes involved. But the fact that the three osteopathic principles have this linkage (different kinds of causes) means that we have discovered a way to connect them and their separate fields of interactions. We now have a *unified* field theory to integrate the interactions *among* these principles and across the mind, body, and spirit.

We probably should not be surprised that Still's principles were related by being types of causes. He was praised for addressing the cause of health problems rather than just treating effects. Philosophy is defined as the study of ultimate causes and so we can say that he was a philosopher. Further, since a unified field theory connects several fields of cause-effect interactions, we can also say that Still was working toward a unified field theory.

Interestingly for those who see healthcare treatment as a type of management, the four basic schools of management have also been shown to align with these four dimensions of cause. Indeed, today's managers are taught that they must use the insights of all four schools of management to truly cover all of the dimensional aspects of management. For instance, while you need objectives or a final cause, you also need processes (efficient cause), good structures (material cause), and overall concepts or formulations (formal cause) to make things happen.

Something's Missing

Do we also need this four-dimensional view of reality in healthcare? Do we need to understand all of the dimensions or aspects of change involved? We have three types of causal principles that explain three of the major overviews of healthcare. We also have a model that explains the continuity (the unified field) among them. Do we need to find a possible fourth dimension of change in healthcare?

The answer is "of course." Surely, healthcare should be as well understood and managed as business. We should be happy that the writings of Aristotle brought this deficiency to our attention. We should also be happy that Aristotle's model indicated what type of causality we missed. What we seemed to have missed in our unified theory of healthcare is related to Plato's **final cause**. Plato believed that things happened or changed because of their final objective or intention. So, what we have theoretically missed has to do with the *objectives* for the changes in disease or health. It may seem strange that objectives would be a part of the natural laws involved in health or disease. Then again, the particular laws of nature under study here deal with people, and people can have objectives.

Summary

This chapter introduced the concepts of field theory and unified field theory using some examples from Albert Einstein. Since field theory was a model to explain many simultaneous cause-effect *interactions*, we decided to further understand the interactions among the mind, body, and spirit before developing a unified field theory for these interactions.

We found that the mind (conscious psychology) could affect the spirit (unconscious psychology), as when the spirit assents to something proposed by the mind, forming a belief. The spirit or belief, in turn, can affect the mind, as when we articulate something based on our confidence in ourselves or consideration of others. We also learned that the spirit can affect the body, as when it activates the body's autonomic nervous system. Conversely, the body's circulatory and nervous systems were shown to affect the mind and spirit.

We expanded on the concept developed in the last chapter that there needed to be healthy "structures" for the mind and spirit, as well as the body, if they were to function well separately or interactively. Further, the principle of *interactive unity* was used to explain why these interactions took place and the principle of *self-healing mechanisms* to explain the formation of defense mechanisms as an example of self-healing in the spirit.

We then explained that the three osteopathic principles could be expanded from principles of the *body* to principles of the *person*, involving the mind, body, and spirit. Next, we showed that these three expanded principles had continuity *among* each other since they were just three different explanations of changes or types of causes:

1. Form(al) Cause — Interactive Unity
2. Material Cause — Structure-Function Interdependency
3. Efficient Cause — Self-Healing Mechanism
4. Final Cause — (Forthcoming)

Lastly, we noticed that there was not a healthcare principle related to a *final* cause. That aspect will be discussed in the next chapter. The search for the final cause or fourth dimension of healthcare changes will involve a quest across several centuries of continuing questions and partial answers. The result will be a startlingly simple solution.

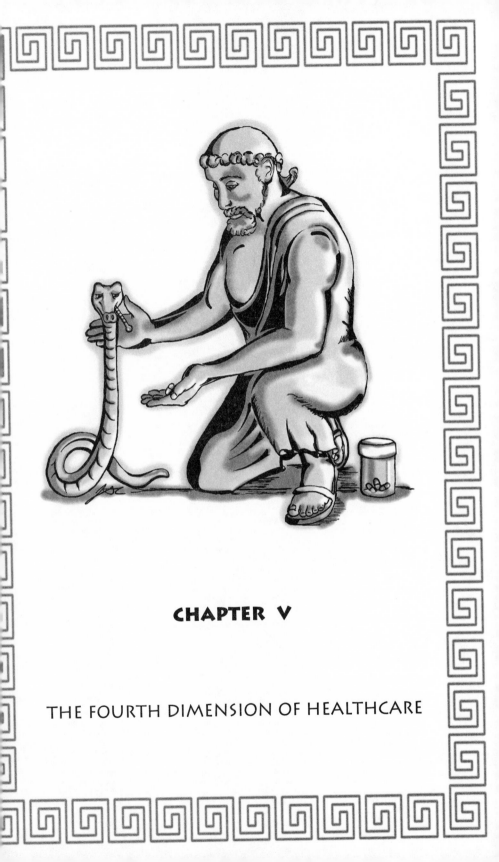

CHAPTER V

THE FOURTH DIMENSION OF HEALTHCARE

THE FOURTH DIMENSION OF HEALTHCARE

Virtually everything we do is to change the way we feel.

—Anthony Robbins

IN ALIGNING the three principles of osteopathy with the four types of causes explained by Aristotle, it appears that one principle has been undetected. Present osteopathic principles do not address Plato's *final cause*, where he believed that things were caused because of the objective or meaning of the change.

Keeping the Objective in Sight

Since an objective is in the mind, this type of cause appears to have something to do with the mind or spirit. We have discussed objectives in the first chapter where we noticed that auto-suggestion played a large part in ancient medicines. Actually, some people today believe all medications are really just a part of the history of placebos.[82]

The placebo effect is usually related to medical research and is defined rather negatively as "an intervention designed to mimic the modality or process being studied."[83] On the other hand, proactive use of the placebo is now being considered to try to cause good results. The positive, therapeutic definition of the placebo effect is "a treatment modality or process administered with the belief that it possesses the ability to affect the body only by virtue of its symbolic significance."[84]

An Active Placebo

While the active use of the placebo concept is supposedly new to the medical arts, its efficacy, under various names, has been reported for a long time. Elmer Lee, M.D., wrote in 1898:

> The principle influence or relation [of drugs] to the cure of bodily disease lies in the fact that drugs supply material on which to rest the mind while other agencies are at work eliminating the disease from the system, and so the drug is frequently given the credit.[85]

While Lee may have put things too strongly, we know today that about one-third of the subjects in a placebo group show a positive response during double-blind research study.[86] The question becomes: Can we somehow *use* the placebo response to get positive therapeutic results?

The large percentage of positive responses from a placebo, combined with the fact that medicines have historically been found to be somewhat ineffective and often to have side-effects, should encourage us to use the placebo approach as much as possible. Howard

Brody, M.D., Ph.D., of Michigan State University has closely studied the positive aspect of the placebo response. Significantly for our formulations, he differentiates between the placebo response and spontaneous healing or self-healing:

> In *spontaneous recovery*, the body goes about its business unaided; no message from our own minds or from other persons' minds comes to stimulate the process. In the *placebo response*, we presume that a message has made an impact on the mind, which then turns on new chemical pathways, or at least accentuates and strengthens the pathways that are already operating.[87]

Brody goes on to say that this prompting of the body to use its own, internal drugstore is a very natural process and empowers the person as a "healer."[88] But, the striking aspect of the above quotation for our present analysis is that it shows that self-healing mechanisms and the placebo response are *different*.

A Different Principle Altogether

The above section indicates that the placebo response is not the same as the self-healing mechanism. Could it be then that the active use of the placebo response is our fourth principle? We know that A. T. Still realized that the nerves which were freed by manipulation signaled the internal drugstore to help various parts of the body. Still also lived among the Native Americans for a short time and clearly appreciated their sense of a pervading spirit throughout all of nature, including the human body. He referred to this spirit as the "inner man," which controlled the actual healing. Therefore, even if vaguely, Still seemed to have had at least a rough sense of how our activated spirit or heightened expectancies could set our inner healing mechanisms in motion. We may now have the needed insights to complete his general inclinations in this regard.

What's in a Name

Today, osteopathic physicians are known for listening to patients. This may explain (via the placebo response) part of their effectiveness. It may now be time to define this aspect of their care as another osteopathic principle.

One key to activating the self-healing and drugs-of-the-body seems to be related to being listened to.[89] Brody asserts: "Telling your story and being listened to and understood may well be a crucial aspect of healing."[90] Besides showing interest, a healthcare professional who is carefully listening is showing serious analysis of the problem and thereby inspires more confidence in the patient about what is recommended:

> If a physician offers me an explanation for my illness, what makes it a *satisfactory* explanation? [emphasis original] It seems reasonable that if he has carefully listened to me, I will have a much higher level of *confidence* that he is explaining *my* illness, and is not simply handing me a stock explanation off the shelf.[91] (emphases added)

In various placebo studies with worthless procedures or inoperative drugs, only the power of the participants' confidence or expectancy can explain the high percentage of success.[92] Even today, with sophisticated double-blind studies, it is hard to prove the superiority of antidepressant drugs over placebos.[93]

The key ingredient for success in these cases seems to be positive expectancy. Brody suggests three aspects of the placebo response: **conditioning, expectancy, and meaning**.[94] He defines conditioning as how what happened in the past affects our inner pharmacy (now).[95] He goes on, however, to cite studies that suggest that conditioning ultimately can be considered a part of expectancy: "Therefore, expectancy accounts for all the observations, leading to the conclusion that if conditioning has any role at all, it works by creating an expectancy that one will feel better after taking a placebo."[96]

On the other hand, meaning does not seem to be included within the expectancy response. Meaning decreases the extent of the illness or pain when one of three types of meaning is present: the illness is explained; care or concern is expressed by another; or enhanced control over the illness seems forthcoming.[97] Meaning develops understanding about the illness. In a general sense, meaning gives an objective to why the illness is happening.

You Make a Difference

The expectancy aspect of the placebo response also gives an objective to the illness in the sense that it helps someone understand what will or should happen. As we have seen, positive thoughts (conscious mind) can affect our unconscious mind (spirit), which controls our autonomic healing system. Brody explains it like this:

> All we are doing, after all, is listing potential linkages that might explain placebo responses. The fact that the immune system undergoes changes attributable to what we think and feel about what is going

on around us, gives us a potential clue to one means by which a placebo response might work. At the very least, instead of thinking the immune system is separate from the effects of the mind, we need to remember that it seems designed specifically to influence and to be influenced by both the mind and the nervous system.[98]

Coupling meaning and expectancy as two independent but related parts of bodily response also points out that individuals should take more credit for their healing. Indeed, this focus on individual response should motivate health practitioners to deliberately try to motivate their patients to develop a "take-charge" attitude to help "stoke up" their inner pharmacy.[99] Thus, developing meaning and expectancy could be a major part of healthcare.

How then do we state these findings as a fourth dimension of healthcare? Since we seem to need both meaning and expectancy, we should call this fourth principle the meaning-expectancy response. Including the word *response* should help physicians and other health professionals remember that their listening and discussion should empower their patients, not just themselves. Disease and health reside *within the patient* and, given this chapter's insights into the response from a patient's understanding and expectancy, patients need to understand that it is their healer within that is most important. In turn, health professionals need to understand that the patient is the star and they have a supporting role.

Summary

This chapter reminded us that ancient medicine often relied on auto-suggestion or what is now called the placebo response. The placebo response was different than self-healing mechanisms and so it became a possibility as the fourth principle of osteopathy. This became all the more appropriate when we realized that osteopathic physicians have a long history of giving their patients a sense of meaning or objective about their treatments. The objectives were what Plato referred to as the *final cause* of change and this cause was one of the four kinds of causes recognized by Aristotle.

Therefore, the placebo response, or what is more descriptively called the meaning-expectancy response, is proposed as the fourth general principle of healthcare. Each of these general principles is just a different aspect of cause:

1. Form(al) (Formulation) Cause — Interactive Unity
2. Material (Structural) Cause — Structure-Function Interdependency
3. Efficient (Process) Cause — Self-Healing Mechanisms
4. Final (Meaning) Cause — Meaning-Expectancy Response

The next chapter examines some of the interactions among the mind, body, and spirit using these four principles. In so doing, we obtain a clearer understanding of how these principles form a unified field theory. The first part of the chapter proposes various characteristics of a unifying theory. The second part provides at least two research findings supporting each of the four principles. Simply put, the first part of the next chapter describes what should be in the unifying theory and the second part describes how the proposed theory meets those criteria.

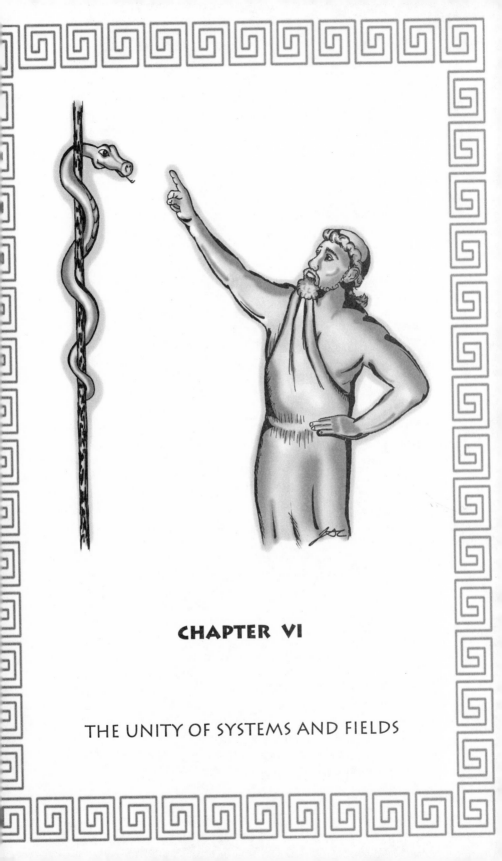

CHAPTER VI

THE UNITY OF SYSTEMS AND FIELDS

THE UNITY OF SYSTEMS AND FIELDS

We know too much and feel too little.
—Bertrand Russell

Now that we have derived the four principles of healthcare, we need to show how they meet the criteria for a unifying theory to coordinate healthcare and how each principle coordinates the interactions among the body, mind, and spirit.

Four Principles of Healthcare

The four principles of healthcare based on Aristotle's types of causes are:

1. **Interactive Unity**. The various parts of a person's mind, body, and spirit are interactive, so disease or health in one part can affect other parts.

2. **Structure-Function Interdependency**. There are interdependencies among structures and functions, where restoring natural structures helps functioning, and various types of func-

tioning can affect structures of the mind, body, or spirit.

3. **Self-Healing Mechanisms**. A person's mind, body, and spirit have natural predispositions toward self-adjusting or adapting to restore natural structures and functioning.

4. **Meaning-Expectancy Response**. A person can bring changes to the responses of the mind, body, or spirit through the expectancy or meaning attached to a stimulus or event.

Of course, the overarching principle of osteopathic care is still valid and should be added to the four causal principles:

5. **Holistic Treatment**. For healthcare to be comprehensive in analysis and hence effective in treatment, all of the above basic principles should be considered during treatment.

These are very general principles that various types of healthcare professionals can use, from physicians and nurses to counselors and social workers. This chapter is not about the individual systems of the body or mind or spirit but about the much less discussed *interactions* among these systems. Since we are talking about many fields of cause and effect, we refer to this kind of analysis among several fields as a *unified field study*.

Characteristics of a Unified Field Study

The study of human systems is only truly useful when we understand how to use this information in treating the whole person. A detailed knowledge of the nervous system, for instance, is useless unless the practitioner knows how it is involved in the life of the patient. This need for an integrated understanding of the person's systems has been urged for decades, but with little result. Stevan Cordas, D.O., M.P.H., addressed this issue in 1983:

> One purpose of this article is to advise primary care practitioners to obtain skills beyond the usual medical curriculum training, in a system, or systems, which permits him to assist the patient in obtaining a more harmonious emotional state. This goal appears to be best accomplished by enlisting a non-authoritarian manner that either allows the patient to share in the responsibility for healing or instructs the patient in a self-help method of practical problem solving.[100]

Impressively, Dr. Cordas also appreciated the proactive use of the placebo effect in that same article: "Instead of the negative connotation accorded the placebo effect in the past, it should be appreciated by the practitioner as a neurophysiologic event related to self-healing and body wisdom [meaning] in keeping with osteopathic theory and practice."[101] Further, he saw the shortcomings of the separate study of related systems:

> Many of us would also segregate functions of the immune system from the functions of the neuro-endocrine system; yet, recent investigations indicate that they are closely linked.
>
> The immune system is immensely complex. It is a constant sentinel dedicated to maintaining the integrity of the individual by discriminating between self and nonself, and mediating between host and pathogen. Yet, increasingly, data indicate that this

system is not totally autonomous and like all physiologic systems functioning in the interest of homeostasis, it is integrated with, and subject to, modulations by the CNS [central nervous system].[102]

Stephen A. Kardos, D.O., a physician with a similarly sounding name, is presently revolutionizing medical education at the founding osteopathic medical school, the Kirksville College of Osteopathic Medicine in Missouri, by introducing real-case studies in learning how several aspects interact in patient care. That is, by studying a patient over time and during several treatments, medical students can learn about the *interactive dynamics* that are a critical component of healthcare. Training should neither be totally static nor one-dimensional, but rather should teach something about the interactive processes among the mind, body, and spirit.

The same call for interactive understanding came in 2001 from W. Llewellyn McKone, D.O., in England:

> Osteopathic principles do not allow systems to be considered separately in clinical practice. Academically three main systems have been brought together in the discipline of psychoneuroimmunology, with the addition of a fourth, the myofascioskeletal system, being the most energetic. . . . In this way we find ourselves back where we started, talking with and examining the patient. For years it has been demonstrated that there is a direct and reciprocal communication between the immune, nervous, and endocrine systems.[103]

Even Robert Ader, M.D., of the University of Rochester (New York), who first used the word *psycho-*

neuroimmunology in 1981, did not think there was a way to teach an inter-systems, interactive approach.

> And when it comes to teaching psychoneuroim-munology, I don't think you can teach the *field* by having a series of lecturers come in and describe their own particular discipline or area of research. That may be a multidisciplinary course; it's not an interdisciplinary course. I have argued for years ... that the disciplines into which science has been divided ... constitute arbitrary and artificial bound-aries that reflect our own intellectual limitations rather than the nature of the biological phenomena with which we are concerned. Psychoneuroimmu-nology is certainly a case in point. We know enough to know that it will not be possible to understand immunoregulatory processes without considering the nature and state of the organism in which immune responses take place. We have as much to learn about neural and endocrine function—and behavior—from the integrated study of immune function as we have to learn about the immune sys-tem from studying it as one component of the inte-grated system of adaptive processes.[104] (emphasis added)

What Ader was saying is that we need to study sys-tems in psychoneuroimmunology by seeing their role with other systems, *not* by studying each system sepa-rately. We need an interfield approach. Ader also said, "We're not talking about the causation of disease, but the **interaction** between psychosocial events, coping and the preexisting biologic conditions."[105] (emphasis added)

The question then becomes how do we conceptual-ize all these interactions for understanding and use?

The proposed solution is to use the four Aristotelian types of causes as dimensions of a unified field theory. This solution is demonstrated in the next four sections.

1. Form(al) Cause (Pythagoras)

The form(al) cause deals with formulations and models, and is related to the osteopathic principle of **interactive unity**. Interactive unity is an overall formulation used to explain *how* things change. Interactive unity was inspired by Rudolf Virchow, who proposed that cells of all types needed to have sufficient nutrition (input) and excretion (output) so that disease in one part did not fester and cause problems in other parts. We expanded that to suggest that health in key parts can help bring health to diseased parts. Then we went beyond these bodily interactions to include interconnections among the body, mind, and spirit.

Cora Barden, D.O., gave perhaps the simplest way to understand this mind-body-spirit interaction:

> It may be that, for various reasons, he does not wish, and therefore has no will [spirit] to get well. Here, too, then, the mind of the patient seems to be a real factor in the success of the cure. Man is not merely a physical machine. He is a complex entity composed of body, mind, and spirit, marvelously interacting in a physico-spiritual unity. . . .[106]
>
> Is not this unconscious the soul [spirit] of man? And is it not the soul what Dr. Still said we must also treat and heal if our healing is to be fully effective? . . . Yet the physician may see only the disease which is but an affect [*sic*] and be totally unaware of the psychic or spiritual cause. . . . With our understanding of the place of the mind itself in healing, this is no mystery. We know it happens, and

we know why it happens: because man is a *unity*, a complex of body, mind, and spirit;...[107] (emphasis added)

Another example of this interactive unity is seen in the following interaction of the mind and spirit. The conscious *mind* somehow can reach the spirit or *will*, which unconsciously controls the autonomic nervous system. To appreciate that, we must realize that the autonomic nervous system has two parts: sympathetic and parasympathetic. During unstressful times, the parasympathetic system runs the autonomic nerves; during stressful times, the sympathetic system takes charge and releases epinephrine (adrenaline) to initiate the fight-or-flight response:

> Given the opposing nature of the two branches, the sympathetic and parasympathetic systems cannot be activated simultaneously. You cannot be stressed out and chilled out at the same time. While it's true that stress cranks up the sympathetic engine, the reverse also is true: Parasympathetic activity turns the sympathetic motor off and pulls the key out of the ignition.[108]

With the "either-or" functional information above, the needed treatment becomes apparent: We should try to turn off the sympathic (stressful) system and turn on the parasympathetic (unstressful) system. But can we do that? Can the mind interact with the spirit? Modern research says "yes" to both questions:

> Most of us think that attitude must change before behavior changes. That's true, but the inverse works too. If you force yourself to behave in a way

that's out of synch with how you actually feel, your brain won't long be able to tolerate the incongruity. It'll change your attitude to come into accordance with your behavior. In psychological lingo, the term is **cognitive dissonance**.[109]

Because of this "either-or" functionality, the *mind* can devise ways to improve the disposition or *spirit*. In turn, the improved spirit then interacts with and improves the operations of the bodily nervous and healing systems.

In this quick evaluation of the "truth" of the **interactive-unity** principle, we found that the spirit can control bodily health and that we can use our minds to develop a healthy spirit. These are illustrations of the way interactivity unity can explain the **how** of causes in healthcare.

2. Material Cause (Thales)

The material cause deals with the material and structures involved and so is related to the osteopathic principle of **structure-function interdependency**. The principle of structure-function interaction was inspired by the work of people like Louis Pasteur and Claude Bernard in controlling the functioning of ecological structures in the body. But what about structure-function interactions between the body and mind or body and spirit?

As we have learned from earlier sections, there *are* interactions among the structures and functions of the body with those of the mind and spirit. The following research finding suggests links between the fields of immunology (related to the body) and psychology (related to the mind and spirit):

Note the correlation between the presence of
cytokines [immune chemical agents] and emotional
[psychological] state. Cytokines show up not only
when we are physically sick but also when we are not
well psychologically.[110]

Thus, the bodily reaction to being physically sick
and psychologically sick is the same!

Researchers have also addressed the interdependency of system structures and functions:

Because of pro-inflammatory cytokines, the
symptoms of having a bad cold and being depressed
are similar. . . . What this means is that in the presence of either a pathogen or severe emotional stress,
the body reacts in virtually the same way. It means
not only that stress can make you ill but also that,
via cytokines and pathogens, your immune system
can stress you out and affect you psychologically.[111]

Therefore, if we view "structures" as systems as well
as bones and other physical structures, we are in a better position to appreciate **what** interdependencies are
operating, even between structures and functions that
cross between mind, body, and spirit.

Robert Sapolski, Ph.D., of Stanford University, provided another example of the interaction between the
mind or spirit and the body in the casual sense of structure and function. Sapolski found that stress, if continued over time, can kill brain cells in an area related to
memory and parts of the brain related to Alzheimer's
disease.[112] This is an example where functioning (with
stress) can cause a change in structure. Usually, we only
think that structures can control functions, not vice

versa, and not between functions of the mind and structures of the body.

To summarize the above study of the **structure-function interdependency** principle of change, we found that the immunologic response to bodily and mental problems can be the same and that problems of the spirit (e.g., stress) can affect bodily cells and structures. These are just two examples of the way structure-function interdependency can explain the **what** of causes in healthcare.

3. Efficient Cause (Heraclitus)

The efficient cause deals with the doers or processes of change, and is related to the osteopathic principle of **self-healing mechanisms**. The self-healing mechanisms were inspired by the work of theorists like Charles Darwin and Herbert Spencer, who maintained that the body had inherent inclinations to improve, to adapt, and to heal. We advanced this view to include the mind and spirit as well as the body.

One of the best descriptions of the efficient causality of self-healing bodily parts has been given by Irvin Korr, Ph.D., of the Kirksville College of Osteopathic Medicine:

> Essentially this role [of the spinal column], speaking figuratively, is that of a "keyboard" through which the brain finds expression. The spinal cord is . . . where most of the . . . nerves emerge; it is where most connections are made between the tissues and organs of the body on the one hand and the central nervous system on the other. About 99 percent of the sensory information from the body itself

is fed into the spinal cord where it receives its first preliminary coding.[113]

The spinal cord is clearly a doer and can be looked upon as the cause of many activities of the body. Therefore, we can understand the spinal cord as an *efficient* cause. Different systems can be understood in different ways; it is just a matter of what kind of cause most clearly illustrates the dynamics involved.

The efficient aspect of causes can also be useful in linking fields of study across the mind, body, and spirit. Once again, Korr provides our example, this time for interfield analysis among the mind, body, and spirit:

> In a healthy person the lesioned [ill-structured or damaged] segment represents a site, a channel, of increased vulnerability. Whether or not disease develops depends upon the other factors in that person and in his life—inherited, developmental, environmental, emotional, social, nutritional, traumatic, microbial, and others.[114]

In this case, Korr is explaining that self-healing mechanisms exist that span across the mind, body, and spirit and so disease development depends on our emotional, nutritional, traumatic, etc., states of healthiness.

In summary, regarding the efficient or **self-healing mechanisms**, we found that the spinal cord can be viewed as a mechanism automatically or naturally orchestrating nerve responses and that disease develops according to the limited functioning or state of healthiness of the various self-healing mechanisms. These are examples of the way **self-healing mechanisms** can explain the **who** or processes of healthcare causes.

4. Final Cause (Plato)

The principle of **meaning-expectancy response** is related to the concept of a final cause. The meaning-expectancy response was inspired by the work of Howard Brody and Roger Bulger, who explained the positive aspects associated with the placebo effect. We further advanced this principle to include the spirit as well as the mind and body.

Esther Sternberg, M.D., the director of the Molecular, Cellular, and Behavioral Integrative Neuroscience Program and chief of the section on Neuroendocrine Immunology and Behavior at the National Institute of Mental Health and National Institutes of Health, gave a far-reaching explanation of the interactions of the emotions (mind) and the immune system (body) related to meaning-expectancy response:

> By blending these two sciences—neurobiology and immunology—we will be able to understand . . . how perceptions of events that are colored by *emotions* can influence different components of the immune response, and ultimately disease. And once we understand that, we can begin to design ways in which modifying our emotional responses might help to prevent or change the course of immune, inflammatory, and infectious diseases.[115] (emphasis added)

Sternberg went on to explain our meaning-expectancy response in terms of the interrelated fields of behavioral science and the nervous and endocrine/immune systems:

Perhaps if we could relearn a new set of associations, turn negative into positive, we could in some sense consciously control our health. Perhaps with practice, we could learn to disconnect the feelings from the events that bring them on—through conscious will, through psychotherapy, through meditation or prayer. It then takes one more step to imagine that the emotions that come attached [structured] or disconnected [unstructured] could trigger the nerve and hormone pathways that could change the immune system and thus our physical health.[116]

This quotation not only indicates that there are interactions among the mind, body, and spirit, but indicates that we can cause changes by using the meaning-expectancy response principle.

In 1990, an article by Roger Bulger, M.D., president of the Association of Academic Health Centers raised the issue of physicians' psychological treatment of their patients in terms of its effects on healing:

Thus the old focus on the patient's faith in the pill seems less an accurate descriptor of the placebo effect than is the patient's faith in the doctor who prescribes the therapy. Our profession would do well to re-emphasize the role of trust in the establishment of the kind of therapeutic relationship that can facilitate an appropriate placebo effect.[117]

Brody goes further and explains that the healthcare practitioner must also develop a sense (spirit) of meaning and expectancy in the patient to unlock his or her inner pharmacy and healing systems.[118]

In this section on the final or **meaning-expectancy response**, we found by using this principle that we *can* influence different components of our immune and nervous systems and that physicians not only need to appreciate their effect on patients, but should know that they can empower patients toward better healing by providing meaning and expectancy during treatments. These two illustrations show that the meaning-expectancy response can help explain another dimension of causes, the **why** in healthcare.

Aspects of Investigation

Each of the above sections used a different word to summarize its type of cause. The last section explained the **why**, while other sections explained the **who, what,** or **how** behind changes in healthcare. These are also the aspects a good detective considers. A detective sometimes finds one aspect easier to understand, and so first tries to unravel that dimension of causation. Nevertheless, a detective almost invariably needs to evaluate the other aspects of change or cause to get the full picture. So too in healthcare we can use these words to help us consider the other principles of our unified field theory.

Just as important as having a unifying theory is having one that is simple and easy to use. The four questions, *who, what, how,* and *why* are "triggers" to remember the four principles of healthcare that should be considered in evaluation and treatment.

To summarize our unified field theory in terms of both the type of cause and the detecting word, the following table is given:

Table III: Dimensions of the Unified Field Theory

Type of Cause	Healthcare Principle	Detecting Word
1. Form(al)	Interactive Unity	How?
2. Material	Structure-Function Interdependency	What?
3. Efficient	Self-Healing Mechanisms	Who?
4. Final	Meaning-Expectancy Responses	Why?

Summary

The first part of this chapter gave some of the characteristics or criteria for an interactive healthcare model to explain processes that spanned across the mind, body, and spirit. People like Stevan Cordas, Llewellyn, McKone, and Robert Ader were quoted as saying that such processes cannot be taught or understood by their separate parts. A model uniting the involved fields of study was needed.

The second part of the chapter illustrated at least two examples of mind-body-spirit interactions for each of the four principles of healthcare from recent research findings. The intention was to demonstrate the extent of the "truth" or strength of our model and principles by giving clear examples of their usefulness in understanding and treatment.

The third part of the chapter summarized the commonality among all four principles, not only in that they are types of causes, but that they are "aspects of investigation," and answered the questions *who, what, how,* and *why* according to the following correspondence:

1. Form(al) Cause   — *How?* — Interactive Unity
2. Material Cause   — *What?* — Structure-Function Interdependency
3. Efficient Cause   — *Who?* — Self-Healing Mechanisms
4. Final Cause   — *Why?* — Meaning-Expectancy Response

The remaining chapters might be called the *denouement* or explanation of how our unified field theory can resolve the apparently contradictory approaches to healthcare. For instance, in the next chapter, we will see how many ancient and modern forms of healthcare can be reconciled when we realize that they just emphasize one or more of the above dimensions of cause.

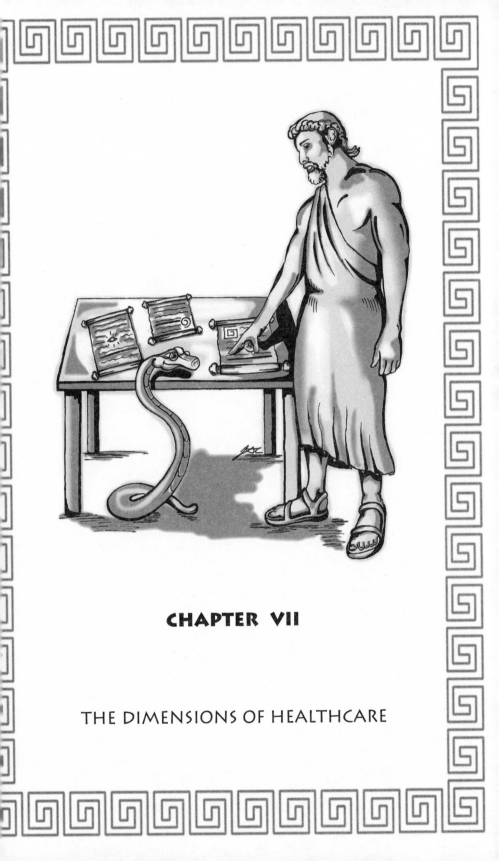

CHAPTER VII

THE DIMENSIONS OF HEALTHCARE

THE DIMENSIONS OF HEALTHCARE

The right word is a powerful agent.
—Mark Twain

WE HAVE all experienced partial success in healing. For instance, we have been able to stop a running nose with decongestants but still have a cold. At other times, we have gotten physically better, but have still remained depressed. These are examples of one-dimensional healing. This chapter examines multidimensional approaches to healing in terms of the proposed principles of healthcare.

Andrew Weil's Spontaneous Healing

One of the clearest books on multidimensional approaches is *Spontaneous Healing* by Andrew Weil, M.D., of the University of Arizona. Weil not only realizes that there are several dimensions of healthcare, but appreciates that they are interactive. For instance, he will not ask a patient to make another attempt to quit smoking until the patient has developed the techniques of stress management.[119]

After talking to Robert Fulford, D.O., Weil stated some principles of healing that closely align with osteopathic principles. His last principle—that the beliefs of practitioners strongly influence the healing powers of patients[120]—aligns with our newly (and independently) added principle of meaning-expectancy response. In other words, Weil believes in the **same** four basic principles of healthcare.

Weil's book includes a series of chapters on "The Faces of Healing," which he describes as follows:

> *[Patients' testimonials about healing]* are testimony to the human capacity for healing. The evidence is incontrovertible that the body is capable of healing itself. By ignoring that, many doctors cut themselves off from a tremendous source of optimism about health and healing.[121]

In one case, Weil explains that doctors simply are not trained to let patients help themselves by using their own internal healing mechanisms: "The patients know better. They want to learn about anticancer foods and supplements, ways of using the mind to boost immune defenses, and so forth."[122] Patients themselves are trying to integrate mind, body, and spirit. Think how much more effective they could be if healthcare professionals explained to them the structure-function interactions or the enhanced response from having meaning and positive expectancy.

Weil also displays an essential sense of the internal self-healing mechanisms:

> I maintain that the final common cause of all cures is the healing system, whether or not treatment is applied. When treatments work, they do so by acti-

vating innate healing mechanisms. Treatment—including drugs and surgery—can facilitate healing and remove obstacles to it, but treatment is not the same as healing. Treatment originates outside you; healing comes from within.[123]

Weil seems to have a fair insight into structure and function and to appreciate, as Still did, that disease is not something external, but an internal problem with a "structure" such as a system:

> Experience with antibiotics and bacteria suggests that exclusive reliance on weapons, however effective they may appear at first, gets us into worse trouble down the road. The weapons themselves influence the evolution of bacteria in the directions of greater virulence, making them more dangerous adversaries. On the other hand, if we concentrate on improving host resistance, the germs stay as they are, and we are protected. So it is probably wiser to rely on the healing system than on drugs and doctors.[124]

In the last few pages, we have seen that Weil agrees with our four principles of healthcare as well as our basic ideas about health and disease. The next sections will review some famous approaches to healthcare and see which of our four principles or dimensions are being addressed. While other approaches could have been selected, these are a cross-section of what exists and can provide a mosaic of how the four principles can be used to explain various dimensions of healthcare.

A. Ayurvedic Healthcare

Ayurvedics is one of the oldest forms of healthcare, going back to the days when philosophers believed in only four elements—earth, air, fire, and water—and in four humors, or bodily fluids, whose balance supposedly determined attitudes. As a result, its teachings may sound very basic to healthcare professionals. However, it has an increasing number of users, perhaps because most regular healthcare practices do not address some important dimensions of healthcare that Ayurvedics addresses.

> [Ayurvedic] practitioners diagnose by observing patients, questioning them, touching them, and taking pulses. With this information the practitioner is able to assign patients to one of three major constitutional types and then to various subtypes. This classification dictates dietary modifications and selection of remedies. Ayurvedic remedies are primarily herbal, drawing on the vast botanical wealth of the Indian subcontinent, but may include animal and mineral ingredients, even powered gemstones. Other treatments include steam baths and oil massages.[125]

Some of the Ayurvedic herbs have been found to be helpful, which is not a surprise, since herbs have been evaluated for many centuries. Its breathing techniques are also useful since, like other breathing approaches, they allow participants to regulate their autonomic nervous system.

Disregarding its belief in previous lives, we can say that Ayurvedics is a continuing, simple system of healthcare that at least appreciates the interactive unity among mind, body, and spirit and the body's self-healing mechanisms. As such, it can offer a few ancient but ever-needed insights. Its limitation, besides its unverified beliefs, lies in its incompleteness and unwillingness to adopt the insights offered by related, scientifically-based research findings. If it does not accept improvements, other approaches will take its good points and thereby eventually supersede Ayurvedics. On the other hand, if it calibrates its ancient teachings in terms of verified findings, it can offer some areas of valid healthcare.

B. Buddhist Healthcare

Buddhism is another ancient approach to living well and has suggested healthcare principles for centuries. An interesting book on the linkages between Buddhism and psychology was written in 2001 by Tara Bennett-Goleman. In *Emotional Alchemy: How the Mind Can Heal the Heart*, Bennett-Goleman provides some excellent insights into the essential aspects of Buddhist teachings: "Buddhism tells us that sometimes a deep insight into the nature of things can come from looking directly, with mindful awareness, at our suffering."[126] Bennett-Goleman asked Erik Kunsang, a translator of Tibetan Buddhism, whether it would be better to concentrate on the spiritual rather than emotional processes. Kunsang said that it was the same process, *dharma*, which had the same meaning as therapy. In this sense, Buddhism and psychological work share the same goal of freeing us from the hold of disturbing emotions.[127] Indeed, the present Dalai Lama, who wrote the foreword of Bennett-Goleman's book, states:

> All such negative thoughts and emotions as hatred, anger, pride, lust, greed, envy, and so on, have the effect of disturbing our inner equilibrium. They also have a taxing effect on our physical health. In the Tibetan medical system, mental and emotional

disturbances have long been considered causes of many constitutional diseases, including cancer.[128]

Bennett-Goleman also explains the important Buddhist concept of *mindfulness*:

> Mindfulness means seeing things as they are, without trying to change them. The point is to dissolve our *reactions* to disturbing emotions, being careful not to reject the emotion itself.[129]

Mindfulness can allow one to change negative emotions into positive emotions. In particular, Buddhism believes in changing the five energies—anger, pride, passion, jealousy, and slothfulness—into sharpness of intellect, equanimity, discriminating awareness, competence, and contemplation, respectively.[130] In general, Buddhism gives a sense of meaning and allows the mind to activate the spirit and thereby calm the systems of the body.

Buddhism addresses some basic needs for emotional stability. It can improve today's psychology with mindfulness and meditation, which can directly calm the autonomic nervous system and help us deal with stress. Buddhism clearly appreciates interactive unity among the mind, body, and spirit, the self-healing mechanisms within and among them, and several aspects of the meaning-expectancy response. As such, it can offer further insights in these three dimensions of healthcare.

Buddhism's liability is that it has not included some sense of the material causes of bodily function, in particular, the interdependency of structure and function. However, it does understand structures in the mind and spirit. Buddhism may have a lot to offer as we strive over the next centuries to apply and further develop the unified field theory preliminarily presented in the four principles of healthcare.

C. Traditional Chinese Medicine

Traditional Chinese Medicine has lasted for many centuries and has over a billion present users. At one time, it was the most advanced form of healthcare and still has several aspects or dimensions involved:

> Diagnosis in TCM [Traditional Chinese Medicine] is based on history, on observation of the body (especially the tongue), on palpation, and on pulse diagnosis, an elaborate procedure requiring considerable skill and experience. Treatment involves dietary change, massage, medical teas and other preparations made primarily from herbs but also including animal ingredients, and acupuncture. The Chinese herbal pharmacopeia is vast, with many plants now under serious scrutiny by Western pharmacologists.[131]

Traditional Chinese Medicine may be the oldest of known healthcare approaches. As such, it has had many centuries to improve, but has limited itself to its traditional dimensions. Like many approaches, it has suffered from a lack of healthy skepticism about itself. That is, it has not tried to find additional dimensions to care for people. However, like other long-lasting approaches, it is a largely unexplored "treasure chest" of insights. Its herbal medicines show promise in such diverse areas as Crohn's disease, chronic bronchitis, sinusitis, osteoarthritis, allergies, asthma, and other autoimmune, infectious, and chronic degenerative disorders.[132]

Traditional Chinese Medicine has many herbs to investigate along with acupuncture and dietary and palpation procedures. It has a general sense of body unity and self-healing mechanisms. Its handicap lies in its rudimentary understanding of body unity and its apparent lack of understanding about structure-function interdependencies and the meaning-expectancy response. Perhaps globalism will encourage Chinese medicine to adopt further dimensions or fields of healthcare as it communicates with other countries and learns more of their practices.

D. Homeopathy

Homeopathy uses very small doses of natural substances to stimulate the immune and other defense systems within the body. There are actually two types being practiced today:

> Classical homeopathy—the kind taught by the founder of the system—specifies the administration of one dose of one remedy selected on the basis of information gained during a lengthy interview with the patient. Nonclassical homeopathy prescribes multiple or regular doses of formulas combining several remedies.[133]

Very diluted doses of substances are supposed to work on the "body's energy field" and "catalyze" the natural healing mechanisms.[134] These terms provide labels rather than explanations. While the homeopathic approach appears to be scientific, close examination shows that it is merely using the external signs of science. It is not based on any research regarding the effectiveness of any dosage, nor related to any known operations of the bodily systems. Lengthy interviews and precise mixtures and dilutions are meaningless if not related to actual structures or functions of the mind, body, or spirit.

In its favor, homeopathy's low dosages most likely do not harm any part of the body. Operationally, it relies on the self-healing mechanisms of the mind and body, and has little else working for it. Therefore, any positive results necessarily come from a placebo effect. Its main limitation is that its procedures are not related to the processes of the body. It could, however, make some progress by testing herbal remedies and working with pharmaceutical companies in double-blind studies.

E. Chiropractic

Although sometimes referred to as a medical practice, chiropractic is not a medical discipline. It does not prescribe medicines (unless over-the-counter relaxants, etc.) and its practitioners are not trained as physicians. Chiropractors use *some* bone-setting aspects that seem related to osteopathic manipulation, but osteopathic physicians believe chiropractic treatments are unsubstantial imitations. More study is needed to sort these claims on both sides.

Chiropractors are well trained in a number of bone-setting techniques and get a great amount of practice by specializing in this one aspect of care. In some cases, where there is an actual obstruction due to a skeletal problem, chiropractors may be able to help the patient. Their treatments are frequently extended over weeks and months and usually include the further costs of many x-rays.

Since chiropractors are not trained as physicians, they may not fully understand the bodily functions underlying their treatments. For instance, many of the previously discussed interactions of the skeletal, nervous, immune, and behavioral systems are not understood or used by chiropractors. The mind-body-spirit interactions are also outside their training. While chiropractors, like other groups, may offer advice on diet, exercise, or nutrition, they do not seem to understand the internal self-healing mechanisms nor the meaning-expectancy principles or dimensions of healthcare.

The worldwide popularity of chiropractic suggests that there is some effectiveness to bone-setting and manipulation. The various users of manipulation, including acupressure, should initiate some ecumenical studies for the good of patients now and in the future. Further, these users need to integrate their practices with the understandings now available from the four principles of healthcare.

F. Naturopathy

In basic terms, naturopathy relies on the curative powers of nature and works to restore the body's own healing ability, using nutrition, herbs, and sometimes homeopathic and traditional Chinese methods.

> Naturopathy comes from the old tradition of European health spas with their emphasis on hydrotherapy, massage, and nutritional and herbal treatment. Older naturopaths may actually be chiropractors with mail-order degrees in naturopathy. Younger naturopaths are well trained in basic sciences and have had exposure to subjects omitted from the conventional medical curriculum, such as nutrition and herbal medicine. Except for their adherence to a general philosophy of taking advantage of the body's natural healing capacity and

avoiding the drugs and surgery of conventional medicine, naturopaths show a great deal of individuality in their styles of practice.[135]

Once again, we see a healthcare alternative becoming popular because of limitations in the range of the dimensions of care practiced by physicians. Natural alternatives are becoming increasingly important as side effects of pharmaceutical drugs and excessive surgery are continuing to be exposed in the media.

Naturopathy's strength rests in its ability to address aspects of healthcare that are seldom addressed by regular physicians and to incorporate natural products and procedures. Naturopathy believes in body unity and self-healing mechanisms and is somewhat comprehensive by addressing several dimensions, including nutrition, exercise, and lifestyle. However, it does not address physiological or psychological effects. Naturopathy's liability lies in its lack of a scientific basis for both its recommendations and its underlying effects on the mind, body, and spirit. It does not address physiological or psychological effects, structure-function interdependencies, or meaning-expectancy responses, which play a significant role in effective healthcare according to recent research.

G. Allopathic Medicine

The term **allopathic medicine** was coined by Samuel Hahnemann in the nineteenth century to separate it from other forms of medicine at that time. Allopathic medicine is the "regular medicine" practiced by M.D.s. Its modern origins in the United States were discussed earlier. While allopathic medical schools apparently do not teach the principles of structure-function interdependency and self-healing mechanisms,[136] they do cover many aspects of interactive unity and some of meaning-expectancy response. In practice, many M.D.s are more interventionists than believers in internal, self-healing mechanisms. Since positive uses of the placebo effect (meaning-expectancy response) have only recently been widely discussed, it is somewhat unfair to criticize any group in that dimension of care. However, the attention informally given to this fourth dimension by osteopathic physicians, Buddhists, and other groups indicates a dimension of care that might well be more widely addressed by allopathic physicians.

The contribution of the allopathic profession lies in its use of the scientific method to detect bodily and mental processes, as well as to develop some seemingly effective drugs. It has great strengths in areas such as surgery, obstetrics, gynecology, ophthalmology, dermatology, pediatrics, radiology, and subspecialties such as oncology. Its practices in these areas should be studied by other healthcare approaches. The limitations of allopathic medicine lie in the neglect of study related to structure-function interdependencies and self-healing mechanisms. In general, allopathic training has little appreciation of any underlying theoretical framework or substratum capable of providing overall, interfield guidance. However, with such a framework, allopathic physicians would be in a strategic position to understand the increasing number of research findings showing interactions among the body, mind, and spirit.

H. Osteopathic Medicine

Osteopathic physicians (D.O.s) are "full service" physicians and do everything that allopathic physicians do, such as deliver babies, perform surgeries, prescribe medicines, and use psychiatric principles. However, osteopathic physicians have an advantage over other healers because of their use of the fundamental principles discussed in this book. Osteopathic physicians use interactive unity to gain a comprehensive sense of how problems in one part of the body can affect other parts, and use structure-function interdependency to understand how poor functioning probably has a corresponding "structural" problem. They use the principle of self-healing mechanisms to understand that every person's bodily, mental, and spiritual systems are doing their best to self-heal. (This belief in individuals doing their best makes them very understanding of people "self-medicating" by alcohol, food, defenses, and other attempts at structuring relief.) Lastly, osteopathic physicians use the principle of meaning-expectancy response (although it has not been previously defined) to provide meaning and encouragement to their patients.

Osteopathic medicine's strength lies in its multidimensional approach to healthcare and its focus on following the natural laws in treatment. Its limitations include the scant research on its principles and practices and its hesitancy in adding valid aspects from other approaches to its recommendations to patients. Osteopathic medical colleges can help by doing research and incorporating the latest scientific findings, teaching valid and useful parts of other approaches, and thoroughly explaining the four overarching principles of healthcare.

Summary

The above approaches addressed different dimensions of healthcare and thereby illustrated the importance of one or more of the proposed principles. Only the osteopathic approach used all four principles, i.e., addressed all four dimensions of healthcare. The strengths and weaknesses of these various approaches to healthcare were discussed to indicate how they could learn from each other and what each could do to improve itself.

The following table gives a rough summary of which dimensions of healthcare were addressed by the approaches discussed above:

Table IV: Approaches and Dimensions of Healthcare

Approach	Interactive Unity	Structure Function	Self-Healing	Meaning-Expectancy
A. Ayurvedics	✓		✓	
B. Buddhism	✓		✓	✓
C. Traditional Chinese	✓		✓	
D. Homeopathy			✓	
E. Chiropractic	✓	✓		
F. Naturopathy	✓		✓	
G. Allopathic Medicine	✓			✓
H. Osteopathic Medicine	✓	✓	✓	✓

The next chapter gives recommendations of ways to use the unified field theory in treatments and discusses how specific treatments use parts of this theory. While the present chapter studied major approaches to healthcare, the next chapter studies very specific treatments and thereby subjects the unified field model to some detailed scrutiny. The results are very revealing not only about the model, but about these well-known treatments.

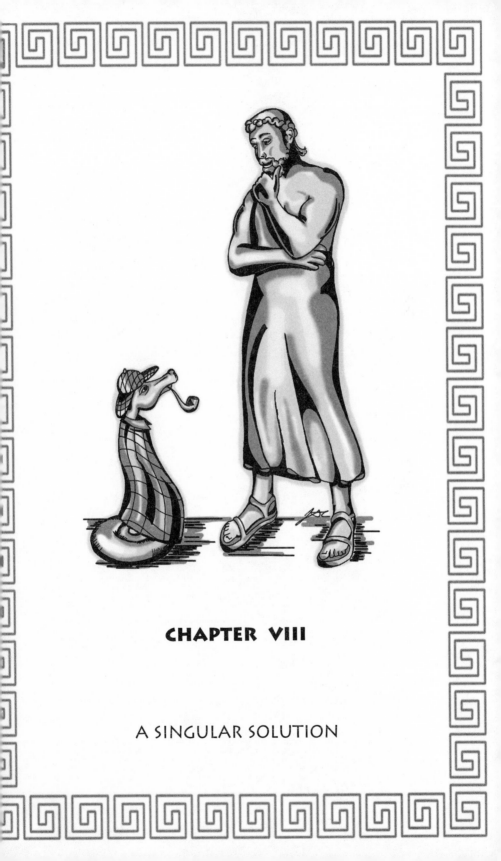

CHAPTER VIII

A SINGULAR SOLUTION

A SINGULAR SOLUTION

We need to change our perspectives, not our problems.

—John Maxwell

ARTHUR Conan Doyle, author of the Sherlock Holmes mysteries, and Gilbert Keith Chesterton, author of the Father Brown stories, both favored the word *singular*. Both detective writers developed clear pictures of facts, and looked to singular traits to help resolve mysteries. Similarly, healthcare practitioners must develop a clear picture of the facts and remember that every case is as unique as the person being studied. Everyone is somewhat different, having various experiences that have arranged the parts of their minds, bodies, and spirits in different ways. Just as A. T. Still and others realized that *disease* was not the germs but the body's response to them, the corresponding point is that *healing* is an individual, internal response.

Individual Response and Dual Development

A doctor's words may encourage you to believe in a medicine or treatment, but only *your* spirit can drive *your* autonomic nervous system to drive *your* internal systems to do the actual healing. That is why, in explaining the meaning-expectancy response, we insisted that it is more important that doctors establish belief *in you* about a treatment than belief *in them.*

Actually, treatment should become a dual development or partnership where the patient and practitioner interact in an integrative process. The patient should change as he or she works with the practitioner, and the practitioner should change by responding to feedback from the patient. As James Gordon, M.D., says in his book *Manifesto for a New Medicine,* "The new medicine is based on a healing partnership in which loving help is given and received and knowledge shared."[137]

A New Picture

The last chapter explained what was missing in regular medicine today and illustrated why the Eastern and alternative types of healthcare were becoming popular. The analysis showed not only the causal perspectives in each of the major approaches to healthcare, but demonstrated the need to have *all* of these perspectives to be truly comprehensive.

The review of approaches across several millennia also reveals the shortcomings of those of recent centuries. In particular, holistic approaches involving the mind or spirit as well as the body are being reintroduced and accepted today because of the natural needs that they fulfill. Western society's movement away from some aspects of religion and belief during the past century has indirectly undermined the use of individual belief or the driving spirit within people in some Western approaches to healthcare.

Today, discussions about a person's motivating spirit or what a person believes about sickness are not usually considered a part of objective healthcare. Instead, our present age focuses on "objective" forms of analysis such as x-rays, CAT scans, and other impersonal assessment procedures. The level of the technology is becoming a surrogate for quality. One contemporary commentator suggested that our present technological approaches to healthcare may be effective in part because of a placebo-type belief in their effectiveness.[138]

In any event, a focus on individuals and a need to work with their spirit and beliefs is at the same time an ancient and yet new approach to healthcare. The unified field theory provides an overview that can include these aspects. An example of the benefits of this kaleidoscopic overview may be demonstrated in how various professionals may now work together:

> This new concept [mind-body-spirit interaction] allows clinical psychologists, psychotherapists, psychiatrists, and primary care physicians to develop integrated insight into the assessment and evaluation of patients with *complex biobehavioral* symptoms. The medical paradigm that emerges is more integrated and holographic (e.g., networked in time/space) than the traditional differential diagnosis and treatment model.[139] (emphasis added)

The unified field theory allows the many aspects of healthcare interactions to come together within one picture, like the matrix of colored pixels allows all the colors present in an object to assemble in their proper places on a computer screen. We need *all* the colors of reality among the pixels if we want to gather all the colors of an object. (Fortunately, the three primary colors, when mixed variously, can form all the colors.) So too, the unified field theory must somehow contain *all* interactions if we are truly to assemble an accurate and comprehensive picture of healthcare interactions among the mind, body, and spirit. (Fortunately, the four principles, when mixed variously, can formulate or describe all the interactions.)

Inside-Out Analysis

We know that relieving peoples' stress can improve their ability to resist getting sick. We also know that the long-term presence of stress can actually make people sick. A brief blood pressure elevation can be positive when it helps individuals survive a physical threat. When prolonged, however, it can cause a stroke. Stress assists the production of the type of cholesterol that clings to the walls of arteries and encourages the destruction of artery-cleaning high density lipoprotein, or HDL. If people have a problem and decide to either fight or flee it, they activate their parasympathetic nervous system and burn the extra sugar in their blood stream, but if they fret undecidedly, they activate their sympathetic nervous system and may develop the symptoms of diabetes.[140]

All of the above adverse developments are very personal and the prevention of their onset depends on each individual's use of systems within their mind, body, and spirit. For instance, are there ways to activate (or deactivate) the autonomic systems? Part of the answer lies in a previously cited quotation:

> You cannot be stressed out and chilled out at the same time. While it's true that stress cranks up the

sympathetic engine, the reverse also is true: Parasympathetic activity turns the sympathetic motor off and pulls the key out of the ignition. A high degree of activity in one system deactivates the other.[141]

In other words, since we cannot be both stressed and relaxed, we can beat being stressed by *deliberately* being relaxed.

The unified field theory supposes that parts of the mind, body, and spirit *can* affect each other, as collaborated by previous citations. The following sections illustrate just a few ways to coordinate these interfield connections. Each example shows different interactions among the mind, body, spirit and thereby illustrates the comprehensiveness of the proposed model.

A. Support Networks

In the recent book *Feeling Good Is Good for You,* authors Carl Charnetski and Francis Brennan point out the importance of support networks:

> The bigger your support network, the better your health, according to numerous scientific investigations. Social support elevates a variety of immune parameters and prolongs survival from the deadliest of afflictions, including heart disease, cancer, and AIDS. Medicine has had solid documentation of the value of social support at least from the 1960s, when Lisa Berkman, Ph.D., from the University of California, Berkeley, compared the health states of more than 7,000 men and women in Alameda County, California, with the extent of their social support.[142]

Social support addresses at least three of the dimensions or types of causes used in healthcare: interactive unity, self-healing mechanisms, and meaning-expectancy response. It also recognizes the mind, body, and spirit interconnections and activates the inner, autonomic, healing systems. As such, social support provides strong multidimensional healthcare. Interestingly, an appreciation of the structure-function interdependency appears to be missing in support networking. The next chapter will point out how this is a promising area for future developments.

B. Music Therapy

While music can calm the savage beast, it can also tame the jungle within:

> Some have theorized that every one of our cells respond, positively or negatively, to different resonant tones. After all, the body does attune itself to certain rhythms. Heartbeat and respiration, for example, tend to synchronize themselves to the best of whatever we happen to be listening to. It's also true that listening to some tunes makes us happy and content, which in turn triggers the body's release of feel-good opioid peptides.[143]

Music addresses three types of causes: interactive unity, structure-function interdependency, and self-healing mechanisms. An interfield sense of what goes on when listening to music reveals that both our minds and spirits are activated, as well as our bodies. Therefore, music can involve your healing mechanisms by calming the nervous system, thereby regulating the connecting systems of the inner body, mind, and spirit. The four interacting principles of the unified field theory can open new vistas for therapy. For instance, upon controlled study, a diet of upbeat music may be found to affect the spirit and hence the functioning of the brain as much as a new drug or extended counseling series on depression.

C. Pet Therapy

Pets have also been shown to have therapeutic value and are increasingly being used to access the inner spirit of people, especially the elderly.

> As a 1999 study at the State University of New York School of Medicine in Buffalo demonstrated, pet owners add, subtract, multiply, and divide better when the animals are present in the room. The study's scientists, according to a 1999 paper delivered in Prague at the Eighth Annual International Conference on Human-Animal Interaction, subjected a group to some mental arithmetic, a known stress inducer. When their pets were with them, the people performed better and reacted more calmly, as evidenced by blood pressure readings and heart rate.[144]

Working with pets uses several of the causes or dimensions of change in healthcare, including interactive unity and self-healing mechanisms, and possibly involves the meaning-expectancy response as well. It also uses the interconnections of the mind, body, and spirit. Once again, our unified field theory suggests that such interactions should be possible. Pets are just another way to help control aberrant functioning in one part by restoring health in another part of an interactive human being.

D. Comic Relief

Norman Cousins believed in his "healer within" and used comic relief to activate his spirit and healing mechanisms in 1964:

> Cousins was diagnosed and handed his 3-month death sentence in 1964, at the age of 39. After reading Hans Selye's groundbreaking research linking stress to health, he decided to go for broke and test the long-held *Reader's Digest* proposition that laughter really is the best medicine. He began a daily diet of Marx Brothers movies, Three Stooges shorts, and episodes of *Candid Camera*. After just 10 minutes of laughing himself silly, Cousins soon notice that he could sleep without pain and without need for medication for up to 2 hours. . . .
>
> More than a decade later, in 1979, a still-healthy Cousins recounted his ordeal and his recovery in the book *Anatomy of an Illness*. . . . He had his last laugh in 1990, when he died at the ripe age of 75.[145]

Comic relief seems to use all the aspects of causality in the area of healthcare. It uses *formulations*, or comical stories, to cause interactions among the mind, body, and spirit. It also uses the *material* of structure-functional interactions, if one considers a happy disposition to be a "structure" that allows for healthy functioning. In turn, it relies on the self-healing mechanisms of the mind, body, and spirit as the *efficient* cause for its desired changes. Lastly, comic relief uses the *final* cause or meaning to develop an upbeat expectancy of having a good response.

In general, comic relief is good "medicine" since it uses all four types of causes or ways of treating healthcare. As such, it is also a good illustration of the efficacy of the multifield model of healthcare proposed in this book.

E. Relaxation Therapy

This section explains three famous approaches to relaxation which will be seen to activate different parts of the interconnected body-mind-spirit human being:

Progressive Relaxation

In the 1920s Dr. Edmund Jacobson pioneered the development of a system called "Progressive Relaxation." ...

He noted that muscles contract at the command of the brain. If the muscles are tense, then the brain is overactive. Overactivity in the brain leads to overdrive in such internal organs as the heart, stomach, and colon. ... To remedy this problem, Progressive Relaxation trainees were taught to tense and then totally relax specific muscle groups.[146]

Autogenic Training

Another perspective on the nature of relaxation can be found in the [1930s] work of Johannes Schultz and Wolfgang Luthe. ... Schultz and Luthe developed a method called "Autogenic Training." With this method, subjects repeated mental directives describing these specific sensations, concentrating on the sensations and thereby creating the autogenic state. Subjects would say to themselves, "My arms and legs are heavy and warm," and focus on feelings of warmth and heaviness in the limbs.[147]

Relaxation Response

Another perspective on the nature of relaxation emerged in the 1970s with the work of Dr. Herbert Benson, a professor at Harvard Medical School. He believed humans to have the capability for a unique and integrated "Relaxation Response." . . . Benson found that specific physiological changes occurred during the relaxation response. These included decreased oxygen consumption, decreased heart and respiratory rate, and a higher proportion of alpha brain waves. These changes represented decreased activity of the sympathetic nervous system. . . .[148]

The above three approaches (**Progressive Relaxation**, **Autogenic Training** and **Relaxation Response**) may be understood in terms of their similarities and differences as illustrated by the four-dimensional causality model. They are similar insofar as they are all self-directed methods for achieving relaxation.[149] They are different in that they approach relaxation from different dimensions or perspectives of causing relaxation.

Progressive Relaxation starts with the muscles of the body expecting to affect the mind or brain and then cause additional relaxation of the inner bodily systems. By tightening and relaxing the muscles, one takes charge of some major bodily functioning and, by interactive unity, one begins to influence autonomic, self-healing mechanisms.

Autogenic Training, on the other hand, starts with the mind expecting to affect the body and, in particular, the autonomic nervous system. By describing specific sensations and concentrating on these sensations, Schultz and Luthe showed that this training induced changes in the controlling mechanism deep in the brain to produce relaxation in the mind and spirit and then in the body. This is an interfield reaction that can easily be understood by the interactive unity, self-healing, and meaning-expectancy principles of the unified field theory.

Relaxation Response also starts in the mind using Benson's four requirements: a quiet environment, comfortable position, passive attitude, and the repetition of a single word. Benson believed this induced state of relaxation reduced the functioning of an overactive sympathetic nervous system.[150] This approach and response can be explained from three different dimensions by the interactive unity, structure-function, and self-healing principles.

Indeed, the five levels of relaxation proposed very recently by John Harvey, M.D., in his book *Total Relaxation: Healing Practices for Body, Mind, and Spirit* need these unified field interactions in order to work. His five levels are: muscular, autonomic, emotional, mental, and spiritual.

In **muscular relaxation**, Harvey uses many of Jacobson's muscular tension release methods, while in **autonomic relaxation**, he uses breathing techniques to get access to the autonomic nervous system: "Breathing slowly and evenly stimulates parasympathetic activation. Consequently, we see that we can use our breathing pattern to achieve autonomic balance."[151]

For **emotional relaxation**, Harvey recommends revising our "self-talks," or what we say to ourselves. He suggests mindfulness and avoiding always-never thinking and all-or-nothing exaggerations. He also suggests talking to a good listener and trying to establish intimacy with another.[152]

For **mental relaxation**, Harvey suggests sensory focusing, similar to Autogenic Training, concentration, and meditation.[153] For **spiritual relaxation**, he suggests prayer, contemplation, and meditation, where the Relaxation Response is helpful.[154] The similar approach to mental and spiritual relaxation occurs because both Autogenic Training and Relaxation Response start with the mind. Harvey does not seem to appreciate the unconscious aspects of the spirit and so his recommendations are similar to those of the mind. However, the unified field theory has pointed out the connections between the spirit and body and so we now know that bodily activities such as deep breathing can relax the spirit.

What is common to all these relaxation approaches is that they use the interactive unity, structure-function, self-healing principles, and meaning-expectancy to improve one area, thereby improving another. Therefore, our model may be able to make some contributions to the area of relaxation. But that is another story.

While this book is focused on the healing mechanisms within individuals, we all recognize that "healers without" are many times needed to trigger an individual's inner mechanisms. The next section suggests some needed traits of these key healers.

Healer Hallmarks

We end this chapter by giving some characteristics of healers and healing models. Since we would like to encourage people to become better healthcare consumers, and health professionals to become better healers, we list Dr. Howard Brody's criteria for picking an integrative healer:[155]

1. Does the healer take the time to explain things?

2. Does the healer tailor the explanation?

3. Does the healer signal to you that questions are welcome?

4. Does the healer seem to care about you as a person?

5. Does the healer help you feel more in control?

6. Does the healer make you feel like a real partner?

7. Does the healer seem to become more powerful as you become more powerful?

8. Does the healer have a sense of humor?

Interestingly, individuals can apply these traits to themselves to see if they are being helpful to the healing processes within them.

Next, we have a quotation from a scientist who is a national expert on neuropsychoimmunologic interactions, but is worried about the present relationship between practitioners and patients. Dr. Esther Sternberg, a section chief at the National Institutes of Health, has the following summary near the end of her book *The Balance Within*, which can serve as the keynote for the new model, or science, of healing:

> The principles underpinning this new science also provide a basis for physicians and health professionals to step back and hear their patients, to recognize that *emotions* do play a very important role in health and disease. And this in turn may help physicians to spend more time listening to what the patient has to say. It may help them think of the

patient as a whole and treat with *words* and with *compassion* before so quickly pushing limb and head and belly through computerized diagnostic tools.[156] (emphasis added)

Lastly, Dr. Roger Bulger suggests that every patient comes to a healing professional in a "quest for mercy."[157] We submit that the *quality of mercy* can be measured in a person's love for others. Mercy or its inner spirit of compassion is given to the extent that professionals believe their patients are akin to themselves, as "other-selves," as people very like themselves and so very likable. Healers, by definition, intrinsically recognize something of themselves in others and so can enter into a healing partnership. Likewise, self-healing requires mindfully liking ourselves, shortcomings included.

Summary

This chapter explained how our unified field theory (of using Aristotle's four causes as a context for the four healthcare principles) is a singular solution because of its emphasis on the *individual* in healing and because it is a *single* paradigm integrating multiple approaches to healthcare. We also believe it is singular because it is *unique* in providing a comprehensive overview for investigation, analysis, and treatment.

The following kinds of treatments were shown to use one or more dimensions of healthcare in explaining interactions among the mind, body, and spirit:

A. Support Networks

B. Music Therapy

C. Pet Therapy

D. Comic Relief

E. Relaxation Therapy

Demonstrating how the unified field theory explains interactions across various fields of study may motivate professionals in one field to use concepts from another. Pointing out how fields like the nervous, immune, and behavioral systems work interactively may encourage more interfield research. Being able to place almost any kind of healthcare treatment in a common context connects them to the "mainstream of healthcare" and thereby should make referral acceptable.

The research cited on the treatments in this chapter shows that we **can** influence our autonomic and other inner systems in several ways. Having a way to understand and treat the interactions among the body, mind, and spirit shows that we **can** take proactive steps to help the healing within human beings.

The last section of this chapter pointed out that, beside understanding the interactions among the systems of a person, we must understand the interactions between the practitioner and the patient. The unified field model is both *interactive* (among systems of the mind, body, and spirit) and *integrative* (between practitioner and patient.) The integrative aspect is based on the "likeness" between the practitioner and the patient. This insight alone suggests a new era in training and treatment. It also suggests attitudes for self-healing.

In the next and final chapter, we will review all our findings and suggest directions for the future. Also, we will see how the proposed model is related to the biopsychosocial model and how cognitive-behavioral theory explains some of the underlying processes within our unified theory of healthcare.

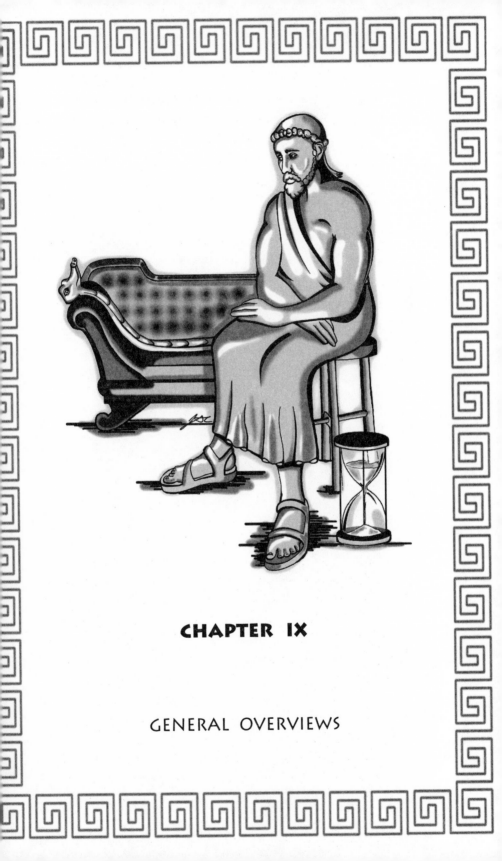

CHAPTER IX

GENERAL OVERVIEWS

GENERAL OVERVIEWS

A good theory is a good learning model.

—Albert Einstein

THE KEY findings of each chapter are provided in the **Review of Findings** below, followed by discussions of the overall processes of healthcare.

Review of Findings

Ancient healthcare contained many important patterns, including auto-suggestion, the effect of attitudes (humors) on health, and models of holistic treatment of the body and mind or spirit. We also saw in the first chapter an appreciation of the relationship between structure and function by Hippocrates and Galen, and an understanding of four types of causes (formal, material, efficient, and final) by Aristotle.

Background was provided in the second chapter on how Andrew Still, in the middle of the United States, took the works of Rudolf Virchow of Germany, Louis Pasteur of France, and Charles Darwin of England to form three very fundamental principles of healthcare:

body unity, structure-function interdependency, and self-healing mechanisms.

Still's comprehensive definitions of **health** (normal structures and functioning) and **disease** (an effect resulting from a disruption of normal structure) were explained. From there, we expanded his principles to include the mind and spirit, explaining that they also had to have orderly "structures" to function well and that they also possessed interactive unity and self-healing mechanisms. The findings of Still, Korr, and Wright emphasized that osteopathic treatments could activate the internal healing mechanisms.

Chapter 4 studied the ways in which the mind and spirit interact (e.g., in forming beliefs) and how the spirit and body interact (e.g., in activating the autonomic nervous system). In studying these relationships, we noticed that they each seemed to cause things to happen from different viewpoints. Interactive unity gives different **formulations** across changes; structure-function interdependency explains the **materials** or structures involved; while the self-healing mechanisms presents the **processes** in the changes discussed. We then realized that these corresponded to three out of the four types of causes explained by Aristotle. This context became the basis of the unified field theory:

1. Form(al) (Formulation) Cause — **Interactive Unity**
2. Material (Components) Cause— **Structure-Function Interdependency**
3. Efficient (Process) Cause — **Self-Healing Mechanisms**
4. Final (Meaning) Cause — (Forthcoming)

The missing principle led to a search for a fourth principle of healthcare based on the final cause, which could explain *why* things happened. A positive type of auto-suggestion or placebo effect, descriptively called the **meaning-expectancy response**, was proposed as a type of final cause. This fourth principle recognized a factor of healing present in ancient healthcare and modern research findings and which was a special characteristic of osteopathic physicians.

Chapter 6 illustrated each of the four healthcare principles in terms of empirical studies. Within these studies, we noticed multiple interactions among the mind, body, and spirit. Indeed, the mind, body, and spirit appeared as **one** field of study because of the many connections and interactions. In a final section on aspects of investigation, we noticed that the four causes actually had a detecting word for each: **how, what, who,** and **why**. Indeed, investigators usually first find one or another aspect of cause easiest to follow but invariably use other aspects to get the full picture.

Chapter 7 explored Ayurvedics, Buddhism, Traditional Chinese Medicine, Homeopathy, Chiropractic, Naturopathy, Allopathic Medicine, and Osteopathic Medicine in terms of how they correspond to one or more of our four dimensions of healthcare. From this overview, we saw that the widely used allopathic medicine only covered two dimensions, which may be why so many people were turning to alternative approaches to get the other dimensions of care. Only osteopathic medicine, when expanded by the addition of the meaning-expectancy response, addressed all four dimensions of causality in healthcare.

Chapter 8 explained how the unified field model was a single paradigm and how it provided a common context for every kind of treatment. The model provided a way to classify (and in some ways evaluate) various treatments. Among the many possibilities, the following specific treatments were analyzed: support networks, music therapy, pet therapy, comic relief, and relaxation therapy. The research cited for each showed that the mind, body, and spirit can indeed influence each other during these treatments, and so such treatments can be connected to "mainstream" healthcare. More importantly, such treatments can reach the inner healing mechanisms and therefore may be used effectively as part of "regular" healthcare.

Further Modeling

The fact that we were able to align some healthcare principles with some types of causes does not mean that there could not be other healthcare principles which could align with these types of causes. Also, the four healthcare principles may each be subsequently found to better correspond to a different cause. In any event, future investigators may be able to use this framework to develop more connections and models.

Using the four types of causes identified by Aristotle does not mean that there can only be four types. In spite of the "authority" of Aristotle, future theorists may be able to develop other types of causes or subcategories, as well as other perspectives on all of the notions discussed.

What about the four healthcare principles themselves? Are they totally independent of each other? Or, as in Isaac Newton's three laws of motion, is one the primary principle and are the others just special cases? We believe the four principles describe different processes and found that they aligned with the four different viewpoints on causality. However, these findings do not preclude finding interactive relationships among these principles.

While many schemes can develop interesting models and theories, they can also be evaluated by their usefulness. In healthcare, this translates into their usefulness in helping people. No doubt, the future of healthcare will be increasingly based on interactive treatments addressing the mind, body, and spirit. Consequently, some form of the unified field theory should become increasingly important. Further, the included osteopathic approach of working with natural processes gives a comprehensive understanding and comprehensive approach to treatments.

Biopsychosocial Model

George Engel, M.D., explained that healthcare needs something beyond the simple biomedical model and the reductionism of the basic sciences. He pointed out that diagnosis also needs to include the psychological, social, and cultural factors.[158] In 1980, Engel proposed the **biopsychosocial model**, which is defined as a systems approach to illness that emphasizes the interconnectiveness of mind and body and the importance of understanding disease at all levels. Engel also said that close attention must be placed on a person's psychological state and the emotional responses to an ongoing treatment.[159]

In many ways, the biopsychosocial model is an attempt at a unified field theory. However, that model delineates **social aspects**, while we choose to delineate the **spirit** as our third part of care. We thought it was important to separate the mind and spirit because of the spirit's key role in activating the internal systems.

We also thought that our **mind-body-spirit model** focuses on the interactions *within* a person and allows the environmental and social aspects to be included *when reacted to* by the person.

The biopsychosocial model uses three of the dimensions of our model in its approach to healthcare: interactive unity, self-healing mechanisms, and the meaning-expectancy response. It does not include the structure-function interdependency and it does not truly use or appreciate the other principles. Further analysis suggests that our unified field theory, based on a mind-body-spirit model, includes all the basic concepts of the biopsychosocial model, but is oriented around health rather than illness.

Nevertheless, biopsychosocial literature is important because it can give further insights into using psychological and social principles in treatments. That is, the literature on the biopsychosocial model is part of what healthcare professionals need to know in order to expand their treatments in the dimensions of the mind and spirit. This is just one example of why health professionals should review existing theories and literature to augment our very general model of healthcare.

Spiritual and Mental Structures

While the **spirit** was involved in treatments in the past, it will play an even larger role in healthcare in the future if it continues to be found to be significant by research. We defined spirit secularly as related to unconscious psychology and distinct from the mind or conscious psychology. In general, spirit is the inner unconscious drives that control some of our mental and bodily functions. However, our healthcare principles suggest that a person's spirit should have a structure if it is to function well. But what is the nature of such a structure? Our model would suggest that even a spiritual structure should be "balanced" like the internal, ecologically balanced structures and systems of the body. That is, we need to have drives, beliefs, etc., that are not unnatural, i.e., not too strong, or eccentric, or unrealizable. The **mind** also needs "balanced" structures as demonstrated by the various attempts at developing responsibility, logic, and social awareness.

Harold Koenig, M.D., Dale Matthews, M.D., and David Larson, M.D., among others, have studied religion as a way to help with depression and other psychological problems.[160] Although they have not referred to religion as a "structure," they suggest that a "spiritual commitment" is very helpful in mental and spiritual functioning. This fits nicely into our proposed mind-body-spirit model and, in particular, into its structure-function principle. For example, a person's religious beliefs can be said to constitute a structure wherein one assesses, assents, and acts in mental and spiritual interactions. The analysis of such structure-function dependencies should be a fruitful area for future developments.

Depression As an Example

To illustrate the comprehensiveness and further expansiveness of the unified field theory of healthcare, we can point to some recent research findings related to our model and principles. Recent research on depression suggests how the mind, body, and spirit are not separate but parts of a single system. The interconnectiveness among these parts unfortunately means that a dysfunction such as depression can make other serious disorders worse. For instance, if you have a heart attack, your risk of dying from cardiovascular disease is four to six times greater if you also suffer from depression.[161] Sometimes depression seems to be an effect rather than a cause: 10% of diabetic men and 20% of diabetic women also have depression, which is twice the rate in the general population.[162] In addition, depression evidently makes people more prone to osteoporosis.[163] Recent studies have also established links between the incidence of depression and cancer, epilepsy, stroke, Alzheimer's and Parkinson's diseases.[164] Depression seems to be a systemic disorder, but that also means that treating it may lessen the severity of other diseases when they occur in the same person.[165]

The theory that the mind, body, and spirit are part of one system (governed by the four healthcare principles) can guide both analysis and treatment. Specifically, the unified field theory suggests treating depression by addressing the spirit, which we now know can be addressed externally by various therapies and religious commitment. In general, it is our hope that the new unifying perspective across mental, bodily, and spiritual interactions will bring increasingly comprehensive understanding and treatment.

Cognitive-Behavioral Concepts

Metacognition is self-awareness or understanding about the cognitive process, or knowing about knowing. This section gives some of the underlying concepts, or metacognition, behind the proposed unifying theory of healthcare.

One can obtain psychological insights into the four healthcare principles by understanding the cognitive-behavioral approach to treatment. We have saved this for last because it can serve as a final culmination of concepts and as a summary of how to proceed with future treatments.

Cognitive-behavioral therapy, which combines the insights of Piaget and Skinner, takes steps to change behavior in terms that will give the client a sense of control and a feeling of hope. It is this reformulation that is the basis of change. Besides developing a hopeful spirit, the therapist tries to form a general context during the initial visit to explore the extent and duration of the presenting problem. During the next step, clients are asked to explore a range of situations where they had comparable thoughts and feelings. During the following step, therapists help clients realize the irrational, self-defeating, and self-fulfilling aspect of their thinking and feeling "structures." (Clients do not usually confront themselves, so a therapist or group is needed to point out the structure causing the poor functioning.) The clients' thinking processes seem to be "stuck" in unhealthy structures of the mind or spirit. The key to unlocking the diseased structures is the confidence in the therapist and in the clients themselves.[166]

The last paragraph implies that there is a process or procedure to follow in order to involve the mind and spirit in healing. Health professionals need to understand this process, at least in a general way, to activate the spirit. This process is important to know because health workers cannot separately treat the body and spirit any more than the neuropsychoimmune system can be understood by separately studying each part.

In a previous section, we explained that we delineated the spirit from the mind because this unconscious part of the psyche activated the inner healing systems. In this section, we saw how cognitive-behavioral therapy explained the process of getting the conscious mind to affect the unconscious spirit. As in a machine, the parts and processes must come together to function properly.

The above insights on procedures suggest that all healthcare healers should have a working knowledge of cognitive behavioral therapy. Otherwise, their attention to bodily functioning, no matter how good, is incomplete. If the theory of mind, body, and spirit interaction is even only partially true, individuals themselves as well as professional healers need to attend to the mind and spirit as well as the body. Fortunately, the unified field theory provides four principles to guide that treatment:

1. **Interactive Unity** explains *how* treating one part of the mind, body, and spirit can help another.

2. **Structure-Function Interdependency** provides guidance about *what* structures control *what* functioning and vice versa.

3. **Self-Healing Mechanisms** explain *who* (what system) does the healing and strongly suggest working with and activating the natural processes.

4. **Meaning-Expectancy Response** tells *why* we should listen to and explain the meaning of disease (unhealthy structure) and work to establish confidence and positive expectancies (healthy functioning) in the client.

Practitioner-Patient Interplay

Ted Kaptchuk, O.M.D., who lectures at Harvard University, believes that the most important thing in the practitioner-patient interaction is "what they pay attention to" when they talk. That is, what things they discuss: is it the bodily data; is it the physical pain; or is it the thoughts and beliefs? Different approaches to healthcare access different components of who we are.[167]

Practitioners need to appreciate the thoughts and beliefs of the patient as well as examine the body. Otherwise, they are only evaluating one dimension of a multidimensional human being. They need to ask: *how, what, who,* and *why.* By addressing all the parts and dimensions of a person, practitioners can bring comfort or peace to the spirit, even when they cannot relieve the bodily pains any further. In this multidimensional approach, practitioners can *reach* the inner bodily and spiritual mechanisms; more than that, they can *activate* the self-healing mechanisms deep inside each individual.

When practitioners are positive, supportive, and best of all, loving, they are not deceiving a patient. They are not using a placebo to fool patients, but rather using the placebo response to bring expectancy, meaning, and best of all, mindfulness. They are ministering to an "other-self," and saying, "I like you, and want to know, help, and empower you." They are saying, "I want to treat your body, mind, and spirit; I want to help you gain meaning, and use your unity, structures, mechanisms, and responses; I want to allow you to access *your healer within.*"

Future Directions

Many areas of future development have been opened by the unified field theory. Although others have suggested that the interactions discussed may be able to happen, our theory singularly laid out a scheme to contemplate and use these interactions in a comprehensive way.

While we tried to make this book an "easy read" by moving the citations to the back of the book, we nevertheless referenced dozens of studies that confirmed the existence of interacting mechanism across the mind, body, and spirit. We are confident that a new era of healthcare is emerging where treatment will be done in an interactive and integrative way.

These recent studies and developments should have large impacts on teaching, research (both theoretical and applied), and on the acceptable practices of all types of healthcare professionals. For instance, healthcare providers will be expected more and more to understand the basic insights of cognitive, behavioral, and biopsychosocial models. Professionals and others will need to realize that the body and mind and spirit are **not** separate systems, and accept new findings in these areas as eagerly as they now look forward to reading about biomedical breakthroughs.

All this is great news for educated adults, who have increasingly felt that there were interactions among the body, mind, and the spirit and that these interactions could help healing. Now they know they can get help in understanding these connections, in validating their uses of "alternative" types of healthcare, and in moving ahead in their strategies for living, learning, and improving.

In more ways than one, this book is a commentary on the human spirit. In the quest for truth, in spite of continuing missteps and comical confusions, the human being remains the world's finest glory and yet greatest mystery.

> Sole judge of truth, in endless error hurled,
> the glory, jest, and the riddle of the world.
> —Alexander Pope

ACKNOWLEDGEMENTS

THE AUTHORS would like to thank the many people who have helped in various ways with this book.

Since the book includes many fundamental concepts learned in classes, the authors would first like to thank their professors at Iona College, Rensselaer Polytechnic Institute, and New York University (for James), and at Adelphi University, the University of Illinois, and Virginia Commonwealth University (for Rene).

The authors are grateful to the many osteopathic and allopathic physicians whom they were honored to learn from and to get to know. In particular, they would like to thank the late Max Gutensohn, D.O., who was a special friend and inspiration. They would also like to thank the executive directors of the American Osteopathic Association (AOA) and the American Association of Colleges of Osteopathic Medicine (AACOM), John Crosby, J.D., and Douglas Wood, D.O., Ph.D., respectively. The AOA and the AACOM jointly sponsored "The Healer Within" exhibit at the Smithsonian Institution in Washington, D.C., from May to September in 2003.

Many of the main contributors to this book, like Andrew Weil, Howard Brody, Irvin Korr, Carl Charnetski, Francis Brennan, John Harvey, Roger Bulger, Esther Sternberg, Ted Kaptchuk, James Gordon, and

Harold Koenig, are still living and their particular contributions are listed in the Endnotes.

At this point we would like to thank Marian Osterweis, executive vice president of the Association of Academic Health Centers, for writing the Foreword.

The next group to acknowledge is the staff of the Still National Osteopathic Museum, starting with its director, Jason Haxton. Cheryl Gracey and Debra Summers come next since they provided over a hundred years of materials on the connections among the mind, body, and spirit, including never published handwritten pages by Andrew Taylor Still.

Jamie Carroll was responsible for the art work on the cover and at the beginning of each chapter.

We received great editorial help from a number of people, including Julie Rosenthal, Susan Nelson, Stacy Tucker-Potter, Jason Haxton, Joan Butt, Ann McEndarfer, Patrice Coughlin, Henry Setser, Danielle Bradshaw, and Nicole McGovern. Breanne Perkins is especially to be thanked for typing and retyping the manuscript and adding helpful suggestions along the way.

Lastly, we would like to thank our families and each other for support and encouragement over many years.

GLOSSARY

ACUPRESSURE Based on the principles of acupuncture, this ancient Chinese technique involves the use of finger pressure (rather than needles) at specific points along the body to treat ailments such as tension and stress, aches and pains, menstrual cramps, or arthritis. Acupressure is also used for general preventive health care.[c]

ACUPUNCTURE In acupuncture, fine needles are inserted at specific points to stimulate, disperse, and regulate the flow of *chi*, or vital energy, and to restore a healthy energy balance.[c]

AIDS (Acquired Immune Deficiency Syndrome) A virus-caused disease that brings about a breakdown in half of the body's immunological defense system.[b]

ADRENALINE (See epinephrine)[b]

ALLERGEN A substance capable of inducing allergy or specific hypersensitivity in a susceptible individual.[b]

ALLERGY A hypersensitive immune state initiated as the result of exposure to a specific allergen. Characterized by exaggerated reactions to substances, the resulting symptoms are most frequently respiratory, dermatological, or gastrointestinal.[b]

ALLOPATHIC MEDICINE Originally coined in the nineteenth century by homeopathic physician Samuel Hahnemann, who used the term to describe medical practice that prescribed drugs with no logical relationship to symptoms, the term is used most often today to distinguish it from alternative modalities such as homeopathy, herbal medicine, etc. Also known as conventional medicine.[c]

ANGIOGENESIS The process by which the body develops new blood vessels. This is triggered by cancerous body cells to produce a blood supply that feeds nutrients to a tumor and thus speeds up its growth.[b]

ANTIBODY These are protein chemical compounds produced by the body to combine with specific foreign substances and render them harmless.[b]

ANTIGEN Any substance that stimulates the immune system to produce an antibody.[b]

ANTIOXIDANT Antioxidants are substances that protect against the oxidation of free radicals, dangerous chemical compounds that promote disease. The vitamins C and E, beta-carotene, and selenium are well-known antioxidants.[c]

ANXIETY A state of mind that involves feelings of fear, apprehension, and uncertainty. It often occurs without apparent external stimulus.[b]

AUTOANTIBODIES An immunoglobulin (antibody) that is formed in response to, and reaction against, a constituent of the tissues of the body that produces it.[b]

AUTOGENIC TRAINING A technique that teaches the body relaxation by means of a form of self-hypnosis. The method directs participants to focus their concentration on specific parts of their bodies with verbal messages.[b]

AUTOIMMUNE Of, relating to, or caused by an immune system that reacts to the presence of an antigen that is part of the body *itself*.[b]

AUTONOMIC NERVOUS SYSTEM The portion of the nervous system concerned with the regulation of the cardiac muscle, smooth muscle tissue, and the glandular system.[b]

AYURVEDIC MEDICINE Practiced in India for more than 5,000 years, the Ayurvedic tradition holds that illness is a state of imbalance among the body's systems that can be detected through such diagnostic procedures as reading the pulse and observing the tongue. Nutrition counseling, massage, natural medications, meditation, and other modalities are used to address a broad spectrum of ailments from allergies to AIDS.[b]

BACTERIA A classification of microorganisms that are typically unicellular. They are non-spore forming and live in soil, water, organic matter, and the bodies of plants, animals, and humans.[b]

BEHAVIORAL MEDICINE A medical discipline that concerns itself with understanding the role of behavior in the genesis of disease and with helping people to control the state of their own health.[b]

BETA-ENDORPHINE A substance (peptide) produced in the brain and released into the body that has powerful pain-killing properties.[b]

BIOFEEDBACK [1]A relaxation technique that uses electronic devices to detect subtle changes in body states by means of sensors.[b] [2]A technique used especially for stress-related conditions such as asthma, migraines, insomnia, and high blood pressure, biofeedback is a way of monitoring minute metabolic changes in one's own body (e.g., temperature changes, heart rate, and muscle tension) with the aid of sensitive machines. By consciously visualizing, relaxing, or imagining while observing light, sound, or metered feedback, the client learns to make subtle adjustments to move toward a more balanced internal state.[c]

BREATHWORK A general term for a variety of techniques that use patterned breathing to promote physical, mental, and/or spiritual well-being. Some techniques use the breath in a calm, peaceful way to induce relaxation or manage pain, while others use stronger breathing to stimulate emotions and emotional release.[c]

CANCER A malignant tumor formed of abnormal body cells that is characterized by the potential for unlimited growth.[b]

CARCINOGEN A substance or agent that incites or produces cancer.[b]

CATECHOLAMINES A group of compounds, including epinephrine and norepinephrine, that have an action similar to that of impulses conveyed by the sympathetic nervous system.[b]

CELL-MEDIATED IMMUNITY One of two general strategies of the body's immune system. This part of the system is responsible for defense against viruses, abnormal cell growth, and certain intracellular parasites.[b]

CHINESE (TRADITIONAL) MEDICINE Oriental medical practitioners are trained to use a variety of ancient and modern therapeutic methods—including acupuncture, herbal medicine, massage, moxibustion (heat therapy), and nutritional and lifestyle counseling—to treat a broad range of both chronic and acute illnesses.[c]

CHIROPRACTIC The chiropractic system is based on the premise that the spine is literally the backbone of human health. Misalignments of the vertebrae caused by poor posture or trauma result in pressure on the spinal nerve roots, which may lead to diminished function and illness.[c]

COMPLEMENTARY MEDICINE Treatments or therapies that complement rather than replace conventional medical (allopathic) practice. Such therapies may include herbal medicine, bodywork, mind/body modalities, etc.[c]

CONTROL GROUP A group of subjects (animals or people) involved in an experimental procedure. They are identical in many respects to another group participating in the experiment, except for the absence of the one factor being studied.

COPING The pattern or methods—defense mechanisms and reactions—used by individuals to deal with stress, both internal and external.[c]

CORTISONE one of the hormones produced in the adrenal cortex. It is largely inactive in the human body until it is converted to cortisol.[b]

CYTOKINE Any of several nonantibody proteins that are released by a cell population on contact with a specific antigen and act as intercellular mediators, as in the generation of an immune response.[a]

DIABETES Diabetes mellitus is a familial constitutional disorder of carbohydrate metabolism characterized by inadequate secretion or utilization of insulin.[b]

ECHINACEA An immune-enhancing herb derived from the ornamental purple coneflower, commonly used to stave off cold or flu symptoms. German research has confirmed echinacea's antiviral and immune-enhancing properties.[c]

ECZEMA An inflammatory skin condition characterized by redness, itching, and oozing lesions that become crusted and hardened. It is usually considered to be at least partially psychosomatic, as are many skin ailments.[b]

ENDORPHIN A substance produced by and released from the brain that acts as a powerful painkiller in the body. The term is derived from *endogenous* and *morphine*. Endorphins also seem to affect learning and memory beneficially and are involved in metabolic and temperature regulation. The amount of endorphins released by the brain is directly related to internal and external stress.[b]

EPINEPHRINE [1]A hormone of the adrenal medulla that is the most potent stimulant of the sympathic nervous system.[a] [2]A catecholamine produced and released by the adrenal medulla in response to stimulation from the nervous system. It is a potent stimulator of the organs regulated by the sympathetic nervous system and may play a role in regulating certain aspects of immune functions. (*Adrenaline* is the British term for epinephrine.)[b]

ESTROGEN A generic term for estrus-producing steroid hormones, one of the female sex hormones. Estrogen is used in oral contraceptives, for treatment of the effects of female menopause, and as a palliative in breast and prostate cancer. It may affect the immune system adversely when present in unbalanced levels.[b]

FASCIA A sheet or band of fibrous connecting tissue binding together muscles, organs, and other soft structures of the body.[a]

FUNGUS Any of a major group of parasitic lower plants that lack chlorophyll. Different types of microscopic fungi can enter the body and cause virulent infections in many different parts and bodily systems, especially when the immune system is suppressed.[b]

GESTALT THERAPY This psychotherapy aims to help the client achieve wholeness (*Gestalt* is the German word for "whole") by becoming fully aware of his or her feelings, perceptions, and behavior. The emphasis is on the "here and now" of immediate experience rather than on the past. Gestalt therapy is often conducted in group settings, such as weekend workshops.[c]

GINKGO BILOBA An extract derived from the fan-shaped leaves of the ginkgo tree, which improves circulation, inhibits blood clotting, and acts as an antioxidant. Research suggests that ginkgo biloba extract may help improve cognitive function in Alzheimer's patients.[c]

HERBALISM An ancient form of healing still widely used in much of the world, herbalism uses natural plants or plant-based substances to treat a range of illnesses and to enhance the functioning of the body's systems.[c]

HERPES A virus-caused skin disease, the symptoms of which are usually clusters of small blisters.[b]

HISTAMINE A substance occurring in the tissues, histamine has two important functions: it causes dilation of the capillaries, which increases capillary permeability and lowers blood pressure; it causes constriction of the bronchial smooth muscle of the lungs.[b]

HIVES A skin reaction marked by the temporary appearance of smooth, slightly elevated patches that are redder or paler than the surrounding skin and that are usually intensely itchy.[b]

HOLISTIC MEDICINE [1]An approach to health whose goal is to treat the entire human being, not just the diseased portion of the patient.[b] [2]Holistic medicine is a broadly descriptive term for a healing philosophy that views a patient as a whole person, not just as a disease or a collection of symptoms. In the course of treatment, holistic medical practitioners may address a client's emotional and spiritual dimensions as well as the nutritional, environmental, and lifestyle factors that may contribute to an illness. Many holistic medical practitioners combine conventional forms of treatment (such as medication and surgery) with natural or alternative treatments.[c]

HOMEOPATHY Homeopathy is a medical system that uses infinitesimal doses of natural substances—called remedies—to stimulate a person's immune and defense system. A remedy is individually chosen for a sick person based on its capacity to cause, if given in overdose, physical and psychological symptoms similar to those the patient is experiencing.[c]

HOMEOSTASIS The normal state of the (adult) body in which it is able to maintain a uniform state of health.[b]

HOPELESSNESS An attitude or state of mind that is despairing, having no expectation of good or success.[b]

HUMORAL IMMUNITY The immunity acquired after the body is exposed to microbial or other antigens. The role of circulating immunoglobulins (antibodies) is most important in this form of immunity.[b]

HYPERTENSION An abnormally high blood pressure and the condition that accompanies the high blood pressure, hypertension can be a symptom of a number of disorders or it can be a primary disease entity (essential hypertension).[b]

HYPERTHYROIDISM Overactivity of the thyroid gland, causing an increase in the basal metabolism and disturbances in the autonomic nervous system. Some types are thought to be psychosomatically involved.[b]

HYPNOTHERAPY A range of techniques that allow practitioners to bypass the conscious mind and access the subconscious, where suppressed memories, repressed emotions, and forgotten events may remain recorded. Hypnosis may facilitate behavioral, emotional, or attitudinal change. Often used to help people lose weight or stop smoking, it is also used to treat phobias and stress and as an adjunct in the treatment of illnesses.[c]

HYPOTHALAMUS The portion of the forebrain that forms the floor and part of its side. It has a role in the mechanisms that activate, control, and integrate peripheral autonomic mechanisms, endocrine activity, and many bodily functions (hunger, body temperature).[b]

IMMUNOLOGY The branch of biomedical science that is involved with the body's response to antigens; the body's ability to recognize "self" and distinguish it from things that are "not self."[b]

INTEGRATIVE MEDICINE Integrative medicine is based on a physician-patient partnership within which conventional and alternative modalities are used to stimulate the body's natural healing potential. This approach to healing neither rejects conventional medicine nor uncritically accepts alternative practices.[c]

KRIPALU YOGA Kripalu yoga uses classical Hatha yoga postures and breathing techniques to help students enter a state of "meditation in motion." Kripalu yoga teachers offer guidance in these yoga techniques and provide an atmosphere in which sensations, thoughts, and emotions can be experienced in safety and relaxation.[c]

LESION [1]A wound or injury. [2]A localized pathological change in a bodily organ or tissue.[a]

LYMPH NODES These are small, rounded bodies that produce lymphocytes to fight invading substances. There are over a hundred lymph nodes distributed throughout the lymphatic system that serve as defense posts for the body against foreign substances causing disease.[b]

LYMPHOCYTES White blood cells that are largely produced by lymphoid tissue and participate in humoral and cell-mediated immunity. T-cells are lymphocytes.[b]

LYMPHOKINES Substances released by lymphocytes that have come in contact with antigens, they are believed to play a role in activating macrophages and cell-mediated immunity.[b]

MACROBIOTICS A low-fat, high-fiber "macrobiotic" diet is based on whole grains, vegetables, sea vegetables, and seeds. A diet of these natural foods, cooked in accordance with macrobiotic principles designed to synchronize one's eating habits with the cycles of nature, is used to promote health and minimize disease.[c]

MACROPHAGES Macrophages are specialized immune cells that engulf invaders and act as scavengers, thereby cleaning them out of the system. Macrophages play a vital role in alerting the immune system to the presence of antigens, both self and nonself.[b]

MASSAGE THERAPY This is a general term for a range of therapeutic approaches with roots in both Eastern and Western cultures. It involves the practice of kneading or otherwise manipulating a person's muscles or other soft tissue with the intent of improving a person's well-being or health.[c]

MASSAGE, SWEDISH The most commonly practiced form of massage in Western countries. Swedish massage integrates ancient Eastern techniques with modern principles of anatomy and physiology. Practitioners rub, knead, pummel, brush, and tap the muscles. Swedish massage is widely practiced, and practitioners vary greatly in their training, technique, and length of sessions.[c]

MEDITATION [1]When used in healing, meditation is a technique in which the subject is taught to relax the body completely and to focus the mind in a way that leads to an altered state of consciousness, one that removes the subject from the usual worries and anxieties of daily life.[b] [2]Meditation is a general term for a wide range of practices that involve training one's attention or awareness so that one's body and mind can be brought into greater harmony. While some meditators may seek a mystical sense of oneness with a higher power or with the universe, others may seek to reduce stress or alleviate stress-related ailments such as anxiety disorders and high blood pressure.[c]

METASTASIZE The process by which a disease spreads from one organ or part of the body to another not directly connected with it. With malignant tumors, this takes place as a transfer of cancerous cells.[b]

MICROBE A minute living organism, either plant or animal. The term is generally applied to bacteria, protozoa, and fungi that cause disease.[b]

MINDFULNESS Moment to moment nonjudgmental awareness. Often spoken of as the heart of Buddhist meditation.[c]

MONOCLONAL ANTIBODIES Antibodies produced in the laboratory from a single clone of cells. These tailor-made antibodies are identical to each other and have greatly increased the scope of immunologic research.[b]

MULTIPLE SCLEROSIS An autoimmune disease in which the nerves of the central nervous system are damaged or destroyed, producing a variety of symptoms such as weakness, lack of coordination, and speech and visual disturbances.[b]

MUSIC/SOUND THERAPIES These therapies use music and/or sound to help clients attain therapeutic goals, which may be mental, physical, emotional, social, or spiritual in nature.[c]

MYOFASCIAL Pertaining to the fascia surrounding and separating muscle tissue.[a]

MYOFASCIAL RELEASE This hands-on technique seeks to free the body from the grip of tight fascia, or connective tissue, thus restoring normal alignment and function and reducing pain. Using their hands, therapists apply mild, sustained pressure in order to gently and frequently stretch the fascia. Myofascial release is used to treat neck and back pain, headaches, recurring sports injuries, and scoliosis, among other conditions.[c]

NATUROPATHIC MEDICINE Naturopathic medicine, a primary healthcare system emphasizing the curative power of nature, treats both acute and chronic illnesses in all age groups. Naturopathic physicians work to restore and support the body's own healing ability using a variety of modalities including nutrition, herbal medicine, homeopathic medicine, and Oriental medicine.[c]

NEUROHORMONES Hormones that either stimulate or are made by the nerves and the nervous system.[b]

NEUROPEPTIDES A neurotransmitter made up of amino acids that is active in the brain or nervous system. Endorphins and enkephalins are neuropeptides.[b]

NEUROTRANSMITTERS A chemical that is discharged from a nerve-fiber ending to carry messages that bring about direct changes in the body's systems. The neurotransmitter is released by one cell and received by another within a fraction of a second.[b]

NOREPINEPHRINE A hormone formed naturally in the body's sympathetic nerve endings. The principal neurotransmitter of that system. (*Noradrenaline* is the British term for norepinephrine.)[b]

OMEGA-3 ESSENTIAL FATTY ACIDS Highly unsaturated fats found in certain types of fish, flaxseed, and other food sources. Research has shown that omega-3s lower the risk of heart attack, reduce inflammation, and possibly help protect against cancer. [c]

OPIATE Any of various sedative narcotics that contain opium or its synthetic derivatives.[a]

OSTEOPATHIC MEDICINE Like M.D.s, osteopathic physicians (D.O.s) provide comprehensive medical care, including preventive medicine, diagnosis, surgery, prescription medications, and hospital referrals. In diagnosis and treatment, they pay particular attention to the joints, bones, muscles, and nerves. They are specially trained in osteopathic manipulative treatment—using their hands to diagnose, treat, and prevent illness.[c]

PARASYMPATHETIC NERVOUS SYSTEM One of the two subdivisions of the autonomic nervous system (the other is the sympathetic nervous system). The parasympathetic nervous system slows the body down and aids in digestion, elimination, and relaxation.[b]

PEPTIDE Any of various natural or synthetic compounds containing two or more amino acids linked by the carboxyl group to one or more amino groups.[a]

PHAGOCYTES A specialized group of white blood cells that is alert to the presence of invader cells or cellular debris and which circulates throughout the body at all times.[b]

PITUITARY A small, oval gland attached to the base of the brain, connected to the hypothalamus by a stalk. Sometimes called the "master gland," the pituitary affects the entire endocrine system through secretion of several hormones.[b]

PLACEBO An inert preparation or substance given to a patient (or group of patients within a controlled experiment) in place of a drug or medicinal substance. It can also be a procedure with no known intrinsic value. In either case, the patient is not informed that what is being given or done is not the prescribed medication or treatment.[b]

PLACEBO EFFECT An improvement in the condition of a sick person that occurs in response to treatment but cannot be considered a result of the specific treatment used.[c]

PROGRESSIVE RELAXATION A relaxation technique developed in the 1930s by Chicago researcher Edmund Jacobson. It requires that the participant concentrate on and consciously relax different parts of the body in progressive order, i.e., the feet, then the ankles, then the calf muscles, etc.[b]

PROTEIN Any of a group of complex organic macromolecules composed of chains of alpha-amino acids.[a]

PSYCHONEUROIMMUNOLOGY The branch of medicine that studies the interrelationships among the mind (psycho), the nervous system (neuro), and the immune system (immunology).[b]

PSYCHOSOMATIC Having to do with the relation of the mind (psyche) to the body (soma). Usually, the term is used to refer to diseases that affect the body but have their origins in emotional or psychological disturbances.[b]

REFLEXOLOGY Reflexology is based on the idea that specific points on the feet and hands correspond with organs and tissues throughout the body. With fingers and thumbs, the practitioner applies pressure to these points to treat a wide range of stress-related illnesses and ailments.[c]

RELAXATION RESPONSE [1]A relaxation technique developed by Harvard Medical School cardiologist Herbert Benson that uses many of the traditional forms of meditation—silence, concentration, and passive states of mind—to achieve deep states of relaxation that measurably affect the body's physiology.[b] [2]The relaxation response occurs through the meditative repetition of a word or short phrase—and the gentle return to this repetition whenever distracting thoughts occur—in order to trigger a series of physiological changes (slowed breathing, heart rate, blood pressure, etc.) that offer protection against stress.[c]

SHIATSU The most widely know form of acupressure, shiatsu has been used in Japan for more than 1,000 years to treat pain and illness and for general health maintenance. Using a series of techniques, practitioners apply rhythmic finger pressure at specific points on the body in order to stimulate *chi*, or vital energy.[c]

SPECIFIC ETIOLOGY The theory that specific diseases have specific causes was first put forth in the sixteenth century; it had no real influence on the practice of medicine until the discovery of "germs" about 100 years ago.[b]

STEROIDS Hormones, many of which are produced by the adrenal cortex. The release of some steroids into the system is governed by the release of ACTH from the pituitary.[b]

STREPTOCOCCUS A strain of parasitic bacteria that takes the shape of a twisted chain. Certain types are extremely pathogenic to humans and animals.[b]

STRESS A vaguely conceived term, usually seen as the response to an outside circumstance or event (stressor), that

leads to turmoil and unrest within a person. This distur-
bance, which is psychological in orgin, leads to physiological
reactions that then cause distress and may lead to disease.[b]

SUPPRESSOR T-CELLS Suppressor T-cells are white
blood cells that inhibit the generation or progression of
immune responses to specific antigens.[b]

SYMPATHETIC NERVOUS SYSTEM The part of the
autonomic nervous system that tends to increase blood
pressure, increase heartbeat, and inhibit glandular secre-
tions, the sympathetic nervous system prepares the body for
fight or flight.[b]

T-CELLS Some of the immune cells that are carried from
their origin in the bone marrow to the thymus gland, where
they are transformed into T-cells. The *T* in T-cells means
"thymus-derived."[b]

THALAMUS The part of the forebrain next to the hypothalamus. It is the relay center for sensory impulses.[b]

TRANSCENDENTAL MEDITATION A relaxation technique based on certain forms of Hindu meditation and
introduced in the West in the late 1960s. Its practitioners
follow a daily discipline of meditation for twenty minutes
twice a day.[b]

VACCINE Dead or weakened pathogenic microorganisms
used as an antigen to produce long-term immunity. A crude
form of vaccination (against smallpox) was practiced in the
Far East centuries ago but did not become a common practice in the West until the nineteenth century.[b]

VAGUS NERVE A major nerve in the body that originates
in the medulla of the brain and continues through the body
into the abdomen. It supplies nerve fibers to the ears,
tongue, pharynx, larynx, and other parts of the body.[b]

VIRUS A group of minute infectious agents without any
independent metabolism. They can only grow and repro-

duce within living cell hosts, which they do by invading the cell and taking over the machinery and materials of the cell itself.[b]

VISUALIZATION A technique that uses the imagination to help patients cope with stress and encourage healing. Patients attempt to heal physical and emotional ailments by imagining positive images and desired outcomes to particular situations. Visualization with the help of a practitioner is known as guided imagery.[c]

WARTS Benign skin tumors caused by a viral infection. They seem to be remarkably susceptible to healing by psychological suggestion.[b]

WHITE BLOOD CELLS Also called leukocytes, these are the basic immune cells of the body and originate in the bone marrow, liver, and spleen.[b]

YOGA Yoga is a general term for a range of mind/body exercise practices used to access consciousness and encourage physical and mental well-being. Some forms concentrate on achieving perfection in posture and alignment of the body; others aim at mental control to access higher consciousness. Between these two are forms of yoga that focus on the interrelationship of body, mind, and energy.[c]

[a] *The American Heritage Stedman's Medical Dictionary.* Boston: Houghton Mifflin Co., 2002.

[b] Steven Locke and Douglas Colligan, *The Healer Within.* Markham, Ontario: New American Library, 1986.

[c] Gail Harris, *Body and Soul.* New York: Kensington Publishing Corp., 1999.

ENDNOTES

Chapter I

1. E. R. Booth, *History of Osteopathy and Twentieth-Century Medical Practice,* rev. ed. (Cincinnati: Caxton Press, 1924), p. 295.
2. Plinio Prioreschi, *A History of Medicine,* vol. 1, *Primitive and Ancient Medicine* (Omaha: Horatius Press, 1995), p. 71.
3. Albert S. Lyons and R. Joseph Petrucelli II, *Medicine: An Illustrated History* (New York: Harry N. Abrams, Inc., 1978), p. 27.
4. Charles Loomis Dana, *The Peaks of Medical History: An Outline of the Evolution of Medicine for the Use of Medical Students & Practitioners* (New York: P. B. Hoeber, 1926), p. 21.
5. Max Neuburger, *History of Medicine,* trans. Ernest Playfair (London: Oxford University Press, 1909), p. 136.
6. Charles Hazzard, *Principles of Osteopathy,* part 2 (Kirksville, Mo.: Journal Printing Co., 1898), p. 63.
7. R. E. Suter, "Hippocratic Thought," *Journal of the American Osteopathic Association* 88 (October 1988): 1251.
8. Dana, *The Peaks of Medical History,* p. 24.
9. Michael Grant, *The Classical Greeks* (New York: Charles Scribner's Sons, 1989), p. 254.
10. Dana, *The Peaks of Medical History,* p. 26.
11. Neuburger, *History of Medicine,* p. 48.
12. Ibid., p. 46.

13. Lois N. Magner, *A History of Medicine* (New York: Marcel Dekker, Inc., 1992), p. 44.
14. Neuburger, *History of Medicine*, p. 57.
15. Ibid.
16. Ibid., p. 58.
17. Ibid.
18. Ibid., p. 59.
19. Ibid., p. 241.
20. Ibid.
21. Ibid., p. 244.
22. Ibid., p. 245.
23. Galen quoted in Neuburger, *History of Medicine*, p. 260.
24. Ibid., p. 253.
25. Neuburger, p. 262.
26. Irvine Louden, ed., *The Oxford Illustrated History of Western Medicine* (New York: Oxford University Press, Inc., 1997), p. 45.
27. Ibid.

Chapter II

28. Benjamin Rush, quoted in E. R. Booth, *History of Osteopathy, and Twentieth-Century Medical Practice*, rev. ed. (Cincinnati: Caxton Press, 1924), p. 312.
29. Ibid.
30. Ibid.
31. Roy Porter, ed., *Medicine: A History of Healing* (New York: Ivy Press, Ltd., 1997), p. 53.
32. Ibid.
33. Ibid.
34. Louis Pasteur, *Germ Theory and Its Applications to Medicine & On the Antiseptic Principle of the Practice of Surgery* (Amherst, N. Y.: Prometheus Books, 1996), p. 108.
35. Ibid., p. 95.

36. Ibid., p. 110.

37. Steven Locke and Douglas Colligan, *The Healer Within: The New Medicine of Mind and Body* (New York: Penguin Books, New American Library, 1986), p. 13.

38. Charles Loomis Dana, *The Peaks of Medical History: An Outline of the Evolution of Medicine for the Use of Medical Students & Practitioners* (New York: P. B. Hoeber, 1926), p. 89.

39. Charles Darwin, *The Origin of Species* (New York: Gramercy Books, 1979), p. v.

40. Ibid., p. 133.

41. Stephen Jay Gould, *The Structure of Evolutionary Theory* (Cambridge, Mass., and London: Harvard University Press, Belknap Press, 2002), p. 1340.

42. A. T. Still, *Autobiography of Andrew T. Still: With a History of the Discovery and Development of the Science of Osteopathy, Together with an Account of the Founding of the American School of Osteopathy*, rev. ed. (Kirksville, Mo.: The author, 1908), pp. 130-31.

43. A. T. Still, *Philosophy of Osteopathy* (1899; reprint, n.p.: Academy of Applied Osteopathy, 1946), p. 4.

44. A. T. Still quoted in Robert E. Truhlar, ed., *Doctor A. T. Still in the Living: His Concepts and Principles of Health and Disease* (Cleveland: Privately published, 1950), p. 123.

45. A. T. Still quoted in George V. Webster, *Concerning Osteopathy: A Compilation of Selections from Articles Published in the Professional and Lay Press with Original Chapter*, rev. ed. (Norwood, Mass.: Plimpton Press, 1919), p. 39.

46. R. E. Suter, "Hippocratic Thought," *Journal of the American Osteopathic Association* 88 (October 1988): 1250.

47. Wilborn J. Deason, "Dr. Still—Non Conformist: How the 'Old Doctor' Reached His Conclusions on

Osteopathy," *The Osteopathic Profession* 1 (August 1934): 24.

48. Ibid., p. 25.

49. M. A. Lane quoted in Webster, *Concerning Osteopathy*, p. 74.

50. G. D. Hulett quoted in Webster, *Concerning Osteopathy*, p. 62.

51. N. E. Harris quoted in Booth, *History of Osteopathy*, pp. 698-99.

52. Carol Trowbridge, *Andrew Taylor Still, 1828-1917* (Kirksville, Mo.: Thomas Jefferson University Press, 1991), p. 185.

53. Deason, "Dr. Still—Non Conformist," p. 26.

Chapter III

54. George V. Webster, *Concerning Osteopathy: A Compilation of Selections from Articles Published in the Professional and Lay Press with Original Chapter,* rev. ed. (Norwood, Mass.: Plimpton Press, 1919), p. 50.

55. H. C. Wallace, "A. T. Still in Baldwin, Kansas," *Journal of American Osteopathic Association* 33 (January 1934): 216.

56. Leon E. Page, *Osteopathic Fundamentals* (Kirksville, Mo.: Journal Printing Co., 1927), p. 145.

57. Webster, *Concerning Osteopathy*, pp. 168-69.

58. Ibid., p. 171-72.

59. Ibid., p. 171.

60. G. B. Andersson et al., "A Comparison of Osteopathic Spinal Manipulation with Standard Care for Patients with Low Back Pain," *New England Journal of Medicine* 341 (4 November 1999): 1465-68.

61. A. T. Still, *Autobiography of Andrew T. Still: With a History of the Discovery and Development of the Science of Osteopathy, Together with an Account of the Founding of the American School of Osteopathy,* rev. ed. (Kirksville, Mo.: The author, 1908), p. 108.

62. R. E. Suter, "Hippocratic Thought," *Journal of the American Osteopathic Association* 88 (October 1988): 1243.

63. I. M. Korr, "Osteopathy and Medical Evolution," *Journal of the American Osteopathic Association* 61 (March 1962): 524.

64. Rene Dubos, *Mirage of Health: Utopias, Progress, and Biological Change* (New York: Harper and Bros., 1959), p. 99.

65. Walther Riese, *The Conception of Disease* (New York: Philosophical Library, 1953), p. 70.

66. Harry M. Wright, "New Perspectives in Medicine: The Role of the Nervous System in Disease," *Journal of the American Osteopathic Association* 62 (August 1963): 1061.

67. Hans Selye quoted in Robert D. McCullough, "Three-Dimensional Osteopathy," *Journal of the American Osteopathic Association* 63 (December 1963): 317.

68. George W. Northup, "Osteopathic Contribution to the Concept of Body Unity (symposium). Psychic Aspects," *Journal of the American Osteopathic Association* 52 (January 1953): 266.

69. Hans Selye, "Stress and Disease," *Science* 122 (October 1955): 625-31.

70. George W. Northup, "Osteopathic Contribution," 267.

Chapter IV

71. Albert Einstein and Leopold Infeld, *The Evolution of Physics: The Growth of Ideas from Early Concepts to Relativity and Quanta* (New York: Simon and Schuster, 1938), p. 221.

72. Ibid., p. 33.

73. Ibid.

74. A. T. Still, "Body and Soul of Man," c. 1902. Andrew Taylor Still Papers, Still National Osteopathic Museum, Kirksville, Mo.

75. Cora Barden, "Practice: Complete Healing of Body, Mind, and Spirit Is Objective of True Osteopathic Physician," *Osteopathic Profession* 18 (February 1951): 34.

76. I. M. Korr, "Sustained Sympathicotonia as a Factor in Disease," in *The Collected Papers of Irvin M. Korr* (Colorado Springs: American Academy of Osteopathy, 1979), p. 78.

77. Barden, "Practice: Complete Healing," 30.

78. Carl Charnetski and Francis X. Brennan, *Feeling Good Is Good for You* (New York: St. Martin's Press, 2001), p. 33.

79. Ibid., p. 38.

80. Ibid., p. 44.

81. Jeffrey S. Bland, "Psycho Neuro-Nutritional Medicine: An Advancing Paradigm," *Alternative Therapies in Health and Medicine* 1 (May 1995): 26.

Chapter V

82. Howard Brody, *The Placebo Response. How You Can Release the Body's Inner Pharmacy for Better Health* (New York: HarperCollins Publishers, Cliff Street Books, 2002), p. 16.

83. Ibid., p. 14.

84. Ibid.

85. Ibid., p. 23.

86. Ibid., p. 29.

87. Ibid., p. 47.

88. Ibid., pp. 47-48.

89. Ibid., p. 88.

90. Ibid.

91. Ibid.

92. Ibid., p. 62.

93. Ibid.
94. Ibid., p. 1.
95. Ibid., p. 56.
96. Ibid., p. 80.
97. Ibid., p. 84.
98. Ibid., p. 127.
99. Ibid., p. 213.

Chapter VI

100. Stevan Cordas, "Emotional Illness," *Osteopathic Annals* 11 (March 1983): 144.
101. Ibid.
102. Ibid., p. 143.
103. W. Llewellyn McKone, *Osteopathic Medicine*, p. 123.
104. Robert Ader, "On the Teaching of Psychoneuro-immunology," p. 319.
105. Robert Ader, quoted in Steven Locke and Douglas Colligan, *The Healer Within*, p. 69.
106. Cora Barden, "Practice: Complete Healing of Body, Mind, and Spirit Is Objective of True Osteopathic Physician," p. 30.
107. Ibid., p. 32.
108. Carl Charnetski and Francis X. Brennan, *Feeling Good Is Good for You*, p. 67.
109. Ibid., p. 55.
110. Ibid., p. 19.
111. Ibid.
112. Ibid., p. 79.
113. Irvin M. Korr, "Vulnerability of the Segmental Nervous System to Somatic Insults," in *The Collected Papers of Irvin M. Korr* (Colorado Springs: American Academy of Osteopathy 1979). Originally published in *The Physiologic Basis of Osteopathic Medicine*. Post-graduate Institute of Osteopathic Medicine and Surgery (1970): 176.

114. Irvin M. Korr, "Andrew Taylor Still Memorial Lecture," in *The Collected Papers of Irvin M. Korr* (Colorado Springs: American Academy of Osteopathy, 1979). Originally published in *The Journal of the American Osteopathic Association* 73 (January 1974): 193.

115. Ester M. Sternberg, *The Balance Within* (New York: W. H. Freeman and Company, 2000), pp. 208-9.

116. Ibid., p. 161.

117. Roger J. Bulger, "The Demise of the Placebo Effect in the Practice of Scientific Medicine—A Natural Progression or an Undesirable Aberration?" *Transactions of the American Clinical and Climatological Association* 102 (1990): 291.

118. Howard Brody, *The Placebo Response: How You Can Release the Body's Inner Pharmacy for Better Health* (New York: HarperCollins Publishers, Cliff Street Books, 2002), pp. 227-28.

Chapter VII

119. Andrew Weil, *Spontaneous Healing* (New York: The Ballantine Publishing Group, 1995), p. 91.

120. Ibid., p. 38.

121. Ibid., p. 53.

122. Ibid., p. 60.

123. Ibid., p. 110.

124. Ibid., pp. 111-12.

125. Ibid., p. 239.

126. Tara Bennett-Goleman, *Emotional Alchemy* (New York: Harmony Books, 2001), p. 251.

127. Ibid., p. 253.

128. Ibid., p. 1.

129. Ibid., p. 6.

130. Ibid., pp. 312-13.

131. Weil, *Spontaneous Healing*, pp. 241-42.

132. Ibid., p. 242.

133. Ibid., p. 244.
134. Ibid.
135. Ibid., p. 245.
136. Ibid., p. 37.

Chapter VIII

137. Roger J. Bulger, "The Demise of the Placebo Effect in the Practice of Scientific Medicine—A Natural Progression or an Undesirable Aberration?" *Transactions of the American Clinical and Climatological Association* 102 (1990): 291.
138. Jeffrey S. Bland, "Psycho Neuro-Nutritional Medicine: An Advancing Paradigm," *Alternative Therapies in Health and Medicine* 1 (May 1995): 24.
139. Ibid., p. 26.
140. Carl Charnetski and Francis X. Brennan, *Feeling Good Is Good for You* (New York: St. Martin's Press, 2001), pp. 69-78.
141. Ibid., p. 67.
142. Ibid., p. 104.
143. Ibid., p. 90.
144. Ibid., p. 125.
145. Ibid., pp. 142-43.
146. John R. Harvey, Ph.D., *Total Relaxation: Healing Practices for Mind, Body, and Spirit* (New York: Kodansha International, 1998), pp. 5-6.
147. Ibid., p. 8.
148. Ibid., p. 9.
149. Ibid., p. 10.
150. Ibid., pp. 9-10.
151. Ibid., p. 70.
152. Ibid., pp. 108-25.
153. Ibid., pp. 136-50.
154. Ibid., pp. 160-74.
155. Howard Brody, *The Placebo Response. How You Can Release the Body's Inner Pharmacy for Better Health* (New

York: HarperCollins Publishers, Cliff Street Books, 2002), pp. 229-33.

156. Ester M. Sternberg, M.D., *The Balance Within* (New York: W. H. Freeman and Company, 2000), p. 206.

157. Roger Bulger, M.D., *The Quest for Mercy* (Charlottesville: Carden Jennings Publishing Co., Ltd. 1998), p. 21.

Chapter IX

158. George L. Engel, "The Need for a New Medical Model: A Challenge for Biomedicine," *Science* 196 (1977): 131-32.

159. George L. Engel, "The Clinical Application of the Biopsychosocial Model," *American Journal of Psychiatry* 137 (1980): 535-44.

160. Dale A. Matthews, Michel E. McCullough, David B. Larson, Harold G. Koenig, Jams P. Swyers, and Mary Greenwold Milano, "Religious Commitment and Health Status: A Review of the Research and Implications for Family Medicine," *Bulletin of the Greene County Medical Society* (July 1998): 47.

161. Michael Lemonick, "The Power of Mood," *Time Magazine* 161, special issue (January 2003): 66.

162. Ibid., p. 67.

163. Ibid.

164. Ibid., p. 68.

165. Ibid., p. 67.

166. Donald Meichenbaum and Myles Genest, "Cognitive Behavior Modification: An Integration of Cognitive and Behavioral Methods" in Frederick H. Kanfer and Arnold P. Goldstein, *Helping People Change* (New York: Pergamon Press, 1980), pp. 408-11.

167. Ted Kaptchuk quoted in interview by Bonnie Horrigan, "Subjectivity and the Placebo Effect in Medicine," *Alternative Therapies* 7 (September/October 2001): 101-8.

BIBLIOGRAPHY

Ader, Robert. "On the Teaching of Psychoneuro-immunology." *Brain, Behavior, and Immunology* 10 (December 1996): 315-23.

Andersson, G. B., Lucente, T., Davis, A. M., Kappler, R. E., Lipton, J. A., and Leurgans, S. "A Comparison of Osteopathic Spinal Manipulation with Standard Care for Patients with Low Back Pain." *New England Journal of Medicine* 341 (4 November 1999): 1465-68.

Barden, Cora. "Practice: Complete Healing of Body, Mind, and Spirit Is Objective of True Osteopathic Physician." *Osteopathic Profession* 18 (February 1951): 20-21, 28-36.

Bennett-Goleman, Tara. *Emotional Alchemy*. New York: Harmony Books, 2001.

Bland, Jeffrey S. "Psycho Neuro-Nutritional Medicine: An Advancing Paradigm." *Alternative Therapies in Health and Medicine* 1 (May 1995): 22-28.

Brody, Howard. *The Placebo Response: How You Can Release the Body's Inner Pharmacy for Better Health*. New York: HarperCollins Publishers, Cliff Street Books, 2002.

Booth, E. R. *History of Osteopathy, and Twentieth-Century Medical Practice*. Rev. ed. Cincinnati: Caxton Press, 1924.

Bulger, Roger J. "The Demise of the Placebo Effect in the Practice of Scientific Medicine—A Natural Progression or an Undesirable Aberration?"

Transactions of the American Clinical and Climatological Association 102 (1990): 285-93.

_____. *The Quest for Mercy.* Charlottesville: Carden Jennings Publishing Co., Ltd., 1998.

_____, and McGovern, John P. *Physician Philosopher.* Charlottesville: Carden Jennings Publishing, Co., Ltd., 2001.

Charnetski, Carl, and Brennan, Francis X. *Feeling Good Is Good for You.* New York: St. Martin's Press, 2001.

Cordas, Stevan. "Emotional Illness." *Osteopathic Annals* 11 (March 1983): 141-47.

Dalai Lama. *Ethics for the New Millennium.* New York: Riverhead Books, 1999.

Dana, Charles Loomis. *The Peaks of Medical History: An Outline of the Evolution of Medicine for the Use of Medical Students & Practitioners.* New York: P. B. Hoeber, 1926.

Darwin, Charles. *The Origin of Species.* New York: Gramercy Books, 1979.

Deason, Wilborn J. "Dr. Still—Non Conformist: How the 'Old Doctor' Reached His Conclusions on Osteopathy," *The Osteopathic Profession* 1:11 (August 1934): 22-25, 44-46.

DiGiovanna, Eileen. *An Encyclopedia of Osteopathy.* Indianapolis: American Academy of Osteopathy, 2001.

Dossey, Larry. *Healing Beyond the Body.* Boston: Shambhala Publications, 2001.

Dubos, Rene. *Mirage of Health: Utopias, Progress, and Biological Change.* New York: Harper and Bros., 1959.

Einstein, Albert, and Infeld, Leopold. *The Evolution of Physics: The Growth of Ideas from Early Concepts to Relativity and Quanta.* New York: Simon and Schuster, 1938.

Engel, George L., "The Need for a New Medical Model: A Challenge for Biomedicine." *Science* 196 (1977): 131-32.

_____. "The Clinical Application of the Biopsychosocial Model." *American Journal of Psychiatry* 137 (1980): 535-44.

Ernst, Ezard, and Harkness, Elaine. "Spinal Manipulation: A Systematic Review of Sham-Controlled, Double-Blind, Randomized Clinical Trials" *Journal of Pain and Symptom Management* 22:4 (October 2001): 879-89.

Gevitz, Norman. *The D.O.'s Osteopathic Medicine in America.* Baltimore: John Hopkins University Press, 1982.

Gordon, Edward E. "The Placebo: An Insight into Mind-Body Interaction." *Headache Quarterly, Current Treatment and Research* 7:2 (1996): 117-25.

Gordon, James G. *Manifesto for a New Medicine.* Reading, Mass.: Addison-Wesley Publishing Company, 1996.

Gould, Stephen Jay. *The Structure of Evolutionary Theory.* Cambridge, Mass. and London: Harvard University Press, Belknap Press, 2002.

Grant, Michael. *The Classical Greeks.* New York: Charles Scribner's Sons, 1989.

Hamburg, Beatrix, M.D., and Hager, Mary. *Modern Psychiatry: Challenges in Educating Health Professionals to Meet New Needs.* New York: Josiah Macy, Jr. Foundation, 2002.

Harris, Gail. *Body and Soul.* New York: Kensington Books, 1999.

Harvey, John R. *Total Relaxation: Healing Practices for Mind, Body, and Spirit.* New York: Kodansha International, 1998.

Hazzard, Charles. *Principles of Osteopathy: Part Two.* Kirksville, Mo.: Journal Printing Co., 1898.

Horrigan, Bonnie. "Ted Kaptchuk, OMD, Subjectivity and the Placebo Effect in Medicine." *Alternative Therapies* 7:5 (September/October 2001): 101-8.

Hrobjartsson, Asbojron, and Gotzsche, Peter. "Is the Placebo Powerless?" *The New England Journal of Medicine* 344:21 (May 2001): 1594-1602.

Kaku, Michio, and Trainer, Jennifer. *Beyond Einstein: The Cosmic Quest for the Theory of the Universe.* Toronto and New York : Bantam Books, 1987.

Kanfer, Frederick H., and Goldstein, Arnold P. *Helping People Change.* Elmsford, New York: Pergamon Press, 1980.

Koenig, Harold G. *Aging and God: Spiritual Pathways to Mental Health in Midlife and Later Years.* Binghamton, N.Y.: The Haworth Pastoral Press 1994.

Korr, I. M. "Andrew Taylor Still Memorial Lecture." In *The Collected Papers of Irvin M. Korr.* Colorado Springs: American Academy of Osteopathy, 1979. Originally published in *The Journal of the American Osteopathic Association* 73 (January 1974): 362-70.

_____. "Osteopathy and Medical Evolution." *Journal of the American Osteopathic Association* 61 (March 1962): 515-26.

_____. "Sustained Sympathicotonia as a Factor in Disease." In *The Collected Papers of Irvin M. Korr.* Colorado Springs: American Academy of Osteopathy, 1979. Originally published in I. M. Korr, ed. *The Neurobiologic Mechanisms in Manipulative Therapy.* New York: Plenum Publishing Corp., 1978.

_____. "Vulnerability of the Segmental Nervous System to Somatic Insults." In *The Collected Papers of Irvin M. Korr.* Colorado Springs: American Academy of Osteopathy, 1979. Originally published in *The Physiologic Basis of Osteopathic Medicine.* Postgraduate Institute of Osteopathic Medicine and Surgery, 1970.

Lemonick, Michael D. "The Power of Mood." *Time Magazine* 161, special issue (January 2003): 64-69.

Locke, Steven and Colligan, Douglas. *The Healer Within: The New Medicine of Mind and Body.* New York: Mentor Books, New American Library, 1986.

Louden, Irvine, ed. *The Oxford Illustrated History of Western Medicine.* New York: Oxford University Press, Inc., 1997.

Leuchter, Andrew F., Cook, Ian A., Witte, Elise A., Morgan, Melinda, and Abrams, Michelle. "Changes in Brain Function of Depressed Subjects During Treatment with Placebo." *American Journal of Psychiatry* 159:1 (January 2002): 122-29.

Lyons, Albert S., and Petrucelli, R. Joseph II. *Medicine: An Illustrated History.* New York: Harry N. Abrams, Inc., 1978.

Magner, Lois N. *A History of Medicine.* New York: Marcel Dekker, Inc., 1992.

Magoun, Harold I., Jr. *Structured Healing.* Vail, Colorado: Author, 2001.

Matthews, Dale A., McCullough, Michael E., Larson, David B., Koenig, Harold G., Swyers, James P., and Milano, Mary Greenwold. "Religious Commitment and Health Status: A Review of the Research and Implications for Family Medicine." *Bulletin of the Greene County Medical Society* (July 1998): 47.

McCullough, Robert D. "Three-Dimensional Osteopathy." *Journal of the American Osteopathic Association* 63 (December 1963): 315-18.

McKone, W. Llewellyn. *Osteopathic Medicine.* Oxford: Blackwell Science, 2001.

Montgomery, Guy H., and Kirsch, Irving. "Classical Conditioning and the Placebo Effect." *International Association for the Study of Pain* 72 (1997): 107-13.

Neuburger, Max. *History of Medicine.* Translated by Ernest Playfair. London: Oxford University Press, 1909.

Northup, George. "Osteopathic Contribution to the Concept of Body Unity (symposium). Psychic Aspects." *Journal of the American Osteopathic Association* 52 (January 1953): 266-69.

Page, Leon E. *Osteopathic Fundamentals.* Kirksville, Mo.: Journal Printing Co., 1927.

Pasteur, Louis. *Germ Theory and Its Applications to Medicine & On the Antiseptic Principle of the Practice of Surgery.* Amherst, N.Y.: Prometheus Books, 1996.

Peck, Connie, and Coleman, Grahame. "Implications of Placebo Theory for Clinical Research and Practice in Pain Management." *Theoretical Medicine* 12 (1991): 247-70.

Porter, Roy, ed. *Medicine: A History of Healing.* New York: Ivy Press, Ltd., 1997.

Prioreschi, Plinio. *A History of Medicine.* Vol. 1, *Primitive and Ancient Medicine.* Omaha: Horatius Press, 1995.

_____. *A History of Medicine.* Vol. 2, *Greek Medicine.* Omaha: Horatius Press, 1996.

Riese, Walther. *The Conception of Disease.* New York: Philosophical Library, 1953.

Selye, Hans. "Stress and Disease." *Science* 122 (October 1955): 625-31.

Slater, R.C. "Osteopathy and Immunity." *Journal of the American Osteopathic Association* 42 (March 1943): 303-6.

Sternberg, Ester M. *The Balance Within.* New York: W. H. Freeman and Company, 2000.

Still, A. T. *Autobiography of Andrew T. Still: With a History of the Discovery and Development of the Science of Osteopathy, Together with an Account of the Founding of the American*

School of Osteopathy. Rev. ed. Kirksville, Mo.: The author, 1908.

_____. "Body and Soul of Man." c. 1902. Andrew Taylor Still Papers, Still National Osteopathic Museum, Kirksville, Mo.

_____. *Osteopathy Research and Practice.* Kirksville, Mo.: Author, 1910.

_____. *Philosophy and Mechanical Principles of Osteopathy.* 1892. Reprint. Kirksville, Mo.: Osteopathic Enterprise, 1986.

_____. *Philosophy of Osteopathy.* 1899. Reprint. N.p.: Academy of Applied Osteopathy, 1946.

Suter, R. E. "Hippocratic Thought." *Journal of the American Osteopathic Association* 88 (October 1988): 1243-46.

Talbot, Margaret. "The Placebo Prescription." *The New York Times Magazine* 6 (9 January 2000): 34-39.

Trowbridge, Carol. *Andrew Taylor Still, 1828-1917.* Kirksville, Mo.: Thomas Jefferson University Press, 1991.

Truhlar, Robert E., ed. *Doctor A. T. Still in the Living: His Concepts and Principles of Health and Disease.* Cleveland: Privately published, 1950.

Vickers, Andrew J., and de Craen, Anton J. M. "Why Use Placebos in Clinical Trials? A Narrative Review of the Methodological Literature." *Journal of Clinical Epidemiology* 53 (2000): 157-61.

Wallace, H. C. "A. T. Still in Baldwin, Kansas." *Journal of American Osteopathic Association* 33 (January 1934): 216.

Webster, George V., ed. *Concerning Osteopathy: A Compilation of Selections from Articles Published in the Professional and Lay Press with Original Chapters.* Rev. ed. Norwood, Mass.: Plimpton Press, 1919.

Weil, Andrew. "Mother Nature's Little Helpers." *Time Magazine* 161:3, special issue (January 2003): 70-71.

_____. *Spontaneous Healing.* New York: The Ballantine Publishing Group, 1995.

Wright, Harry M. "New Perspectives in Medicine: The Role of the Nervous System in Disease." *Journal of the American Osteopathic Association* 62 (August 1963): 1057-63.

_____. *Perspectives in Osteopathic Medicine.* Kirksville: Kirksville College of Osteopathic Medicine, 1976.

INDEX

ABOUT THE AUTHORS

JAMES J. MCGOVERN, PH.D., is the president of A. T. Still University, which includes the Kirksville College of Osteopathic Medicine, the international School of Health Management, the Arizona School of Dentistry and Oral Health, and the Arizona School of Health Sciences. He was previously a physics professor, a member of the clergy, associate director of two state boards of higher education, director of the Office of Health Finance for the State of Illinois, and a vice president at the Medical College of Virginia and at Case Western Reserve University. He is the husband of Rene.

Ph.D., *New York University*

M.S., *Rensselaer Polytechnic Institute*

B.S., *Iona College*

RENE J. MCGOVERN, PH.D., is an associate professor in the Department of Neurobehavioral Science at the Kirksville College of Osteopathic Medicine of A. T. Still University, and adjunct assistant professor in the Departments of Psychiatry, Neurology, and Psychology at Case Western Reserve University. She has lectured and published on different aspects of the interactions of the mind, body, and spirit and is presently the director of the 1.67-million-dollar Elderlynk Project, which provides a rural mental health model for elderly care in ten counties.

Ph.D., *Virginia Commonwealth University*

M.S., *Virginia Commonwealth University*

M.A., *University of Illinois*

B.A., *Adelphi University*